7-day
detox

change your eating habits for life

lesley ellis

foulsham
LONDON • NEW YORK.•TORONTO • SYDNEY

foulsham

The Publishing House, Bennetts Close,
Cippenham, Berkshire SL1 5AP, England

ISBN 0-572-03083-5

Neither the editors of W. Foulsham & Co. Ltd nor
the author nor the publisher take responsibility for
any possible consequences from any treatment,
procedure, test, exercise, action, or application of
medication or preparation by any person reading or
following the information in this book. The
publication of this book does not constitute the
practice of medicine, and this book does not
attempt to replace any diet or instructions from
your doctor. The author and publisher advise the
reader to check with a doctor before administering
any medication or undertaking any course of
treatment or exercise.

Printed in Great Britain by Creative Print & Design (Wales), Ebbw Vale.

CONTENTS

INTRODUCTION

Do you wake up each morning rested, refreshed and raring to go? Are you full of energy and enthusiasm for the best part of your waking day? Or do you spend much of your time feeling a bit like a limp rag, weary and under the weather from the moment you get up in the morning?

If you are in the second category (and you'd be surprised at how many people are) no doubt you are asking yourself why on earth you feel like this. You get enough sleep, you eat enough food, there is no medical problem that your doctor can identify, so why should you feel under par?

Perhaps it is not such a mystery if you look at the way most of us live our lives. We keep hectic, demanding schedules; we leave little time for rest and relaxation; we expose ourselves to noise, anxiety and stress; we eat nutritionally poor-quality food and we chivvy ourselves into keeping going by dosing up the eyebrows with toxic substances such as caffeine, tobacco and alcohol.

Not only that, but our systems have to cope with the flood of preservatives and other chemical additives in our foodstuffs as well as the cocktail of toxins in our environment. Frankly, it is no small wonder so many of us feel off colour. Under this tremendous accumulated bombardment, our poor bodies naturally respond by becoming sluggish and out of sorts.

We can do something about this state of affairs, however. If we change the sorts of foods we put into our bodies and adjust our lifestyles, we can eliminate the overload to our systems. That way our natural energy levels start to return and we begin to feel healthier, fitter and happier.

And that is what a detox programme is all about.

ALL ABOUT DETOXING

Detoxing is the process of cleansing your overworked system and helping it to function more efficiently.

Do you need to detox?
When your system is overloaded, your body responds with a range of symptoms, such as:
- Indigestion
- Feelings of bloatedness
- Belching
- Constipation
- Nausea
- Headaches
- Poor complexion
- Poor-quality hair – dry, brittle or lank
- Persistent fatigue
- Poor concentration
- Minor infections such as cold sores and mouth ulcers
- Irritability
- Depression
- Poor-quality sleep at night

If you are all too familiar with some or all of these symptoms, then detoxing might be the answer.

Check with the doctor
Before you go on any diet, or radically change your eating habits, you should, of course, first make sure that it is the right diet for you. If you are pregnant, or have recently given birth, or are breast-feeding, you should speak to your doctor before starting any kind of different eating routine. Similarly, if you are under medical supervision for a condition, taking any prescribed or non-prescribed medicine, or know you have a medical condition, you should check with your doctor first.

Finally, if you are recuperating from an illness or are in any way worried about your health, do ask for medical advice before starting a different diet.

Once you have the all-clear, you can begin.

How to detox

At the heart of any detox programme is excellent-quality, highly nutritious fresh food. When you detox, you leave processed convenience foodstuffs strictly on the supermarket shelf, and instead eat lots of fresh, natural whole foods – cereals such as rice, millet and buckwheat, whole, unprocessed fruit and vegetables, nuts and seeds, beans and pulses.

This means, for a start, you are greatly increasing your intake of valuable natural fibre. Fibre is that all-important part of the food that your body does not digest, but which helps to get your digestive system working efficiently by carrying waste products out of your system.

The detox programme means you are changing to a diet rich in vitamins and minerals to help repair damage and improve your general, all-round health. By avoiding processed foods, which are generally packed with sugar, salt and artificial additives, you are also cutting out any extra toxic burdens on your system.

At the same time as changing to a better-quality, higher-fibre diet, detox nutritionists also advise making sure you eat lots of the foods they call the natural cleansers – foods such as wholegrain rice, apples, beetroot (red beet), garlic, grapes, onions and carrots. These, they tell us, help to speed up the cleansing process.

While you are following the diet, you should also be drinking plenty of fluids to help wash through your system and eliminate toxins and waste.

Diet alone, of course, is not enough. As well as changing what you eat, you need to support your detox programme in your daily life by giving yourself more good-quality rest, more positive relaxation and more regular exercise – there are tips on how to do this on pages 24–5.

Is it difficult to keep to?

For most people, a detox programme means making definite changes to the way they eat, and these may feel a little peculiar at first. Most of us are creatures of habit, especially when it comes to eating and drinking, so breaking with the accustomed ways of doing things is bound to feel strange.

Once you have started the diet, however, you will soon realise that detox eating is surprisingly easy, enjoyable, varied and, above all, delicious, with a multitude of interesting textures and flavours to explore. In fact, if you are a good-food fan, you will quickly discover that the detox diet is – metaphorically at least – a piece of cake!

No limits

Another major advantage of the detox diet is that you need never be hungry. This is not an eating programme that limits the amount of food you eat in any way. This diet is not about will-power or endurance or deprivation. If you are hungry while you are on the detox diet, you should eat; eat enough to feel properly satisfied. If you become peckish between meals or in the evening, you should give yourself a snack. You need never deprive yourself of food while you are on this programme, but you must always make sure that what you eat is the right kind of food for detoxing (more details about this are on pages 17–23).

You may find that because you are unaccustomed to the bulky, satisfying nature of meals made from natural foods, the portions recommended in the recipes are too big and you cannot comfortably eat the amount suggested. That's fine. Simply eat the amount that is right for you; respond to your body's particular needs. Remember, everybody has different nutritional requirements and, indeed, an individual's needs may change over time, depending on their circumstances.

It is important to become sensitive to your body's needs, and to eat accordingly. In fact, you will probably find that once you start the detox diet, you will naturally become much more attuned to your body's proper individual requirements, not only in terms of how much you need, but also as to the kind of foods your body requires.

Losing weight

You may find you lose a little excess weight when you follow the detox programme. This is nothing to be concerned about. Slimming is not the specific aim of the diet, but if you do gently shed a pound or two of unwanted ballast, don't worry. Just enjoy it as a bonus, and a sign that your system is getting back to its proper balance. Indeed, if you keep up some of the good eating habits after you finish your detox diet, you will probably find those excess pounds will not return, unlike weight lost through faddish slimming diets which tends to pile right back on again as soon as you start eating normally.

If you are already very slim and find yourself losing weight because of the detox programme, you probably need to increase your intake of energy-rich foods. Make sure, for example, that you have regular snacks of highly nutritious foods such as unsalted mixed nuts, bananas, avocados and olives (well rinsed) and non-dairy milk shakes flavoured with fresh fruit juice, nuts and perhaps a little honey.

How much work is involved in the diet?

Because the detox diet includes lots of raw, natural foods, you can decide for yourself how much time you are going to spend preparing your meals while you follow the programme.

Some days, you will probably enjoy spending a leisurely time in the kitchen creating a lavish feast of carefully crafted dishes. At other times you can just throw together a huge mixed salad of fabulous fresh ingredients, or a glorious dish full of ripe fragrant fruit – the result will be delicious and good for you either way. The detox programme is flexible; the choice is yours.

SIMPLE PRINCIPLES OF THE DETOX DIET

There are five simple principles to the detox diet, so understanding and keeping to it is really easy. These five principles can be summed up as:

- **Fresh:** all food must be eaten as fresh as possible.
- **Raw and lightly cooked:** much of your food must be eaten uncooked or only lightly cooked.
- **Whole and natural:** all food must be unprocessed, unrefined, and without artificial additives.
- **Fluids:** you must drink 1.75 litres/3 pints of fluid every day.

- **Detox super-foods:** detox nutritionists recommend including these natural cleansers in your diet every day.

So what is the purpose of these five principles, you might ask, and how do I carry them out?

Fresh foods

The rule about fresh food is essential. While you are on your detox programme, you need to eat foods that are rich in vitamins and minerals. Fresh fruit and vegetables provide some of the best sources of these.

Food quickly loses its nutrients if it is kept too long. Vitamins A, B and C, for example, all disappear from foods kept in strong sunlight – just think of all that vitamin C that is draining away, hour by hour, from the oranges that you piled up in a bowl on your kitchen windowsill!

Some vitamins also disappear from food when they come into contact with the air, which is why it is important to cut and prepare fruit and vegetables immediately before using them. Do not be tempted to do the chopping in advance.

Unfortunately, some vitamins are lost as soon as fruit and vegetables are picked, and this disappearing act continues all the time they are being stored. Many nutrients may have been lost from your 'fresh' fruit and vegetables before they reach the shops. This is why it is important to buy fruit and vegetables in season whenever possible. Out-of-season produce has either been stored since harvest, or has travelled to reach your food shop. Either way, it has probably lost important nutrients in the process.

You can help ensure the freshness of your food if you:
- Buy little and often; don't stock up on produce.
- Always buy the best possible quality; never opt for end-of-sell-by-date special offers, or anything that looks old and sad and wilted.
- Buy local produce if it is available, especially from the farm gate, as you will know it has not been languishing for days on the back of a truck.

- Pick your own from PYO farms, or best of all, grow your own produce – that way the delay between harvest and plate is cut down to minutes, rather than days.
- Buy produce in season.
- Store all fruit and vegetables, except bananas, in the fridge until you need them. This slows down vitamin loss enormously. Cool, crunchy apples and chilled, juicy oranges, peaches and strawberries also make sumptious summer foods.
- Keep other foods in cool, dry, dark conditions; flours, nuts and seeds should be sealed in airtight containers.
- Buy frozen produce rather than canned if you cannot get hold of fresh. Produce that is frozen immediately after harvest and kept at low freezer temperatures maintains much of its goodness. Do not keep it too long in your freezer, and use it immediately it is defrosted.

Raw and lightly cooked
Cooking destroys much of the vitamin content of food. Green vegetables, for example, lose up to 70 per cent of their vitamin C when they are cooked, and this loss is increased if the food is then kept hot after cooking.

You need optimum nutrition when you are on a detox programme, so you should aim to eat as much of your diet as possible raw, or only lightly cooked. That way you not only maximise the nutrient content of your food but also make sure you are supplying your system with plenty of that all-important fibre. (There are some foods, that should only be eaten cooked, of course, specifically dried beans and pulses, rhubarb and potatoes.)

If your digestion is delicate when you first start the detox programme, and you find some foods such as cabbage, cauliflower and other members of the brassica family hard to digest, eat only small quantities raw. If even small amounts disagree with you, eat them cooked. Don't be a martyr to the 'raw' principle! Older people especially find some foods difficult to cope with raw. Don't eat anything raw that causes wind, stomach upsets or discomfort. Hard-to-digest foods may be best eaten at breakfast or lunchtime rather than in the evening when your digestion is slowing down for the night.

Certain herbs and spices are useful in helping make foods more digestible (for more details on this, see page 22).

When you are cooking vegetables, remember that steaming is better than boiling – vitamins are washed away from vegetables swimming in water (which is a good reason for not soaking vegetables in water before cooking). Make sure you cook vegetables until they are only just tender, no more. Test them as they cook, rather than relying on a prescribed cooking time. Different varieties of potatoes, for example, cook at very different rates. Baby vegetables generally cook more quickly than full-grown specimens. Some vegetables such as green beans can be served barely cooked so they are still really quite crunchy.

As soon as your vegetables are at the point of being just cooked, drain them and plunge them briefly under cold running water to stop further cooking and help retain colour, texture and nutrients.

Whole and natural

Whole foods are foods that have not been refined and processed. Refining and processing foods robs them of important vitamins, minerals, enzymes and fibre. Wholegrain rice is better than refined white rice, for example, because refined rice has lost most of its thiamin (vitamin B_1) as well as important fibre during the polishing process which turns it from brown to white. While you are on a detox programme you should aim always to eat whole, unprocessed foods.

Eating whole foods means not peeling fruit and vegetables unless absolutely necessary. Potatoes, for example, need never be peeled, especially if they have been organically grown. Roasted potatoes are delicious with a crisply cooked skin, and unpeeled mashed potatoes are good too – the tiny flecks of skin dotted through the creamy white mash add flavour, texture and of course fibre to the dish.

You should wherever possible buy (or grow your own) organically raised produce. That way you can be sure you are not eating residues of toxic pesticides and poisonous herbicides. Organic food is, admittedly, more expensive than food produced the agro-chemical way, but remember that you will not be wasting any of the organic variety by peeling or scraping – you can eat every bit. It is not always possible to buy organic, however, and it is better to make sure you are eating a good range of really fresh food than to insist on consuming only organic food and finding you are left with one sad swede (rutabaga) to last you the whole week.

If you are relying on non-organic fruit and vegetables, there are some simple precautions you can take. Peel or at the very least scrub them extremely thoroughly. I usually remove the outer leaves of non-organic lettuces and cabbages. Non-organic carrots should be prepared by scraping, then removing the top 2.5 cm/1 in where the chemical residues are concentrated.

Avoid processed foods – they almost always include artificial additives such as colourings, flavourings and preservatives. They also contain astonishing amounts of added sugar, salt and processed fats, all of which you should avoid while you detox.

You should not be eating any added sugar – white or brown – while you detox. Sugar is an almost 'empty' food. It provides energy but nothing else – no fibre, no vitamins, no minerals. Sugar can also encourage unwanted bacteria and yeasts to grow in your gut. And finally, because sugar is very pure energy food, it can upset your body's natural blood sugar levels – when you eat it, it is absorbed too quickly into your bloodstream, causing a short rush of energy to the body, then a low-energy dip.

Getting used to a diet without sugar is not easy, especially if you are used to munching biscuits, cakes and chocolate bars. You may find that going without sugar gives you a headache for the first day or two as your blood sugar levels rebalance. It is important to make sure you keep your energy levels up during this time by eating snacks – a handful of fresh dates, perhaps, or a banana. Do not allow yourself to get hungry. You will find that your body and your tastebuds soon adjust, so that you gradually feel you need less and less sweetness in your food. Indeed, highly sweetened stuff will then start to taste quite revoltingly sickly!

Banning sugar means not using it in cooking. For very sour fruits such as blackcurrants, you may want to add a very little cold-pressed organic honey or natural fruit juice concentrate (available from health food stores) to make them more palatable. Many fruits become quite sweet if you allow them to ripen properly. Ripe bananas, for example, are an excellent source of natural sweetness, as are fresh dates and dried apricots. Try mixing sweeter fruits with tarter varieties.

You should cut your salt intake down to an absolute minimum, too. Cut out all salty foods and avoid cooking with salt as far as possible. Be aware that some foods such as olives (even when well rinsed) and soy sauce contain salt, so should be eaten only in moderation. In very hot climates, however, a little extra salt in the diet may be necessary to help the body retain enough fluid.

Fluids

While you are detoxing, it is important to drink at least 1.75 litres/3 pints of fluid every day to help flush through your system properly. That is about eight mugs or tumblers. And in hot weather you should drink rather more than this.

Eight tumblers might seem like an awful lot of liquid but, in fact, many of us drink much less than our bodies really need because we have learnt to ignore our bodies' thirst signals. When you detox you are returning your body to its natural balance and learning to respond to your body's needs.

Little and often is a good rule to follow, and you will soon get used to drinking the full 1.75 litres/3 pints a day. Start with a glass of hot water when you wake up in the morning, or one of the early-morning wake-up drinks suggested on pages 38–9. These are especially good for getting the system working.

You can then easily make up the rest of your allocation of fluid by spreading it throughout the day. For example, you could have a glass of juice with your breakfast and juice or herbal tea mid-morning. At lunchtime you could choose clear, unsalted stock or herbal tea, and more juice as an energy booster mid-afternoon. You could then have a cup of herbal tea or clear stock at around teatime, followed by a hot drink or juice during the evening and perhaps a glass of hot water or soothing herbal tea last thing at night.

You can drink all kinds of herbal teas while you are detoxing – mint and chamomile are soothing after meals and in the evening, fruit and spice mixtures are warming on a cold day, while nettle tea is considered an excellent cleanser. You can make your own or buy commercially prepared tea bags, but do make sure shop-bought varieties do not contain caffeine, artificial additives or added sugar.

Water is also an ideal drink for detoxing; chilled still and sparkling mineral waters can be especially refreshing – there is a huge range available these days, but make sure you do not buy brands with added artificial flavourings.

Fresh fruit juices are also perfect detox drinks – you can make your own using a blender or juicer (see pages 53–7 for recipes) or buy freshly squeezed juices from the chiller cabinet of the supermarket. Do not keep fresh juice for more than a day or two.

Drinks to avoid when detoxing include alcohol of all kinds, coffee (including decaffeinated), tea, cocoa and drinking chocolate, all sweet fizzy drinks, squashes and cordials except those made entirely from concentrated fruit juices without added sugar or other additives.

Clear broths and stocks make a pleasant change, but make sure they are not salty and do not contain artificial additives. A home-made vegetable stock (see page 15) will keep for two days in the fridge, and is useful for cooking as well as hot drinks. You can use any vegetables you like, but remember that potatoes will make your stock cloudy, cabbage will give it a very pronounced flavour, and beetroot (red beet) will turn it deep pink.

Clear Vegetable Stock

10 ml/2 tsp cold-pressed extra virgin olive oil

2 large onions, chopped

2 large carrots, chopped

1 parsnip, chopped

1 small piece of swede (rutabaga), chopped

2 celery sticks, chopped, plus celery leaves

900 ml/1½ pts/3¾ cups water

2 bay leaves

1 large mixed bunch of fresh herbs – parsley, thyme, rosemary, marjoram, coriander (cilantro)

8 peppercorns

Soy sauce, fresh lemon juice and freshly ground black pepper, to taste

1 Heat the oil in a large saucepan, then add the chopped vegetables.

2 Sauté the vegetables until softened but not coloured, then add the water and bring to the boil.

3 Add the bay leaves, the bunch of herbs, tied together, and the peppercorns, then simmer for about 30 minutes.

4 Strain and taste. You may want to add a little soy sauce or a few drops of lemon juice or some freshly ground black pepper at this point. If the stock is not well flavoured, pour it back into the saucepan and simmer until it is reduced by about a half and taste again.

Detox superfoods

Detox nutritionists tell us that some foods are especially beneficial for cleansing the system. I have listed these below and it is recommended that you eat one or two of these cleansers every day.

- **Round wholegrain rice** is a highly absorbent food, full of vitamins and fibre, that almost never creates an allergic reaction in people. Try to buy organic rice. If you cannot find round wholegrain rice (available from most health food stores) use a brown long-grain variety. Do not use white rice. Boiled wholegrain rice is soothing to the digestive system and a traditional cure for diarrhoea.

- **Beetroot** (red beet) is considered by detox nutritionists to be one of the best vegetable cleansers, helping the digestive system to work efficiently, and flushing through the system.

- **Apples** and **pears** are high in fibre and pectin so they help to clean the intestines.

- **Papayas** and **pineapples** contain fibre, vitamins and minerals as well as useful enzymes to help digestion.

- **Lemons** are not only full of vitamin C but also have strong cleansing effect, and help kick-start the digestive system.

- **Sea vegetables** and **edible seaweeds** are packed with vitamins and minerals, and are extremely soothing to the digestive system. Some kinds of seaweed, such as kombu, are considered especially useful for mopping up toxins in the system and flushing them out.

- **Onions** and **garlic** are valued by detox nutritionists for their antiseptic properties, for boosting the immune system and for their blood-cleansing attributes.

- **Olive oil:** recent scientific research has shown that cold-pressed extra virgin olive oil is good for the heart and blood. It also stimulates the digestive system.

- **Chilli peppers** and other **hot spices** stimulate the digestive system and mucous membranes and encourage the body to flush out wastes and toxins. If your digestive system is delicate and if you are not used to eating spicy foods, use only a little at first.

- **Ginger** is considered an excellent cleanser and extremely calming to the digestion.

WHAT TO EAT

There are seven main categories of foods you should include in your detox diet:
- Fruit and vegetables
- Grains
- Pulses, nuts and seeds
- Oils
- Tofu, fish and chicken
- Dairy and non-dairy produce
- Herbs and spices

Fruit and vegetables

Fresh fruit and vegetables are at the heart of your detox diet, providing much of the fibre, vitamins and minerals that are important for cleansing your system. Almost all fresh fruit and vegetables are valuable additions to a detox diet. Try to buy organic varieties.

Dried fruits should be eaten only in small quantities while you are detoxing, and you should make sure you use an unopened, freshly bought packet. Do not be tempted to dig out a sticky, antiquated box that has been languishing in the back of your food cupboard for months.

The following fruit and vegetables are especially useful for detoxing:
- Apples
- Apricots – fresh and unsulphured dried, available from health food stores; not the bright yellow variety
- Asparagus
- Globe artichokes
- Aubergines (eggplants)
- Bananas and plantains
- Beans – broad (fava), runner, green and fine
- Beetroot (red beet)
- Broccoli
- Cabbage
- Carrots
- Cauliflower
- Celery
- Courgettes (zucchini)
- Cress, rape, mustard and other growing salad plants

- Cucumbers
- Dates – fresh
- Fennel
- Garlic
- Grapefruit
- Grapes
- Kiwi fruit
- Lemons and limes
- Lettuce, rocket, lambs' lettuce, dandelion and other salad leaves
- Melons
- Onions and spring onions (scallions)
- Oranges, satsumas, tangerines and mandarins
- Papaya
- Parsnips
- Peaches and nectarines
- Pears
- Peas
- Peppers (bell peppers)
- Pineapples
- Plums
- Potatoes
- Sea vegetables of all kinds – fresh and dried
- Squash
- Strawberries, raspberries and other berry fruits
- Swede (rutabaga)
- Sweet potatoes and yams (remove the skins)
- Turnips
- Watercress

Grains

Whole grains are essential in your detox diet because they provide energy, fibre and a range of important vitamins.

Wholegrain, or brown, rice is considered the best grain for detoxing. Eat some every day if you can. Try it in savoury and sweet dishes; as a side serving instead of potatoes; as wholegrain rice flour (useful for thickening sauces); as puffed rice or rice flakes (good for muesli and porridge); and as crispy rice cakes which provide tasty substitutes for bread and crackers.

Other useful cereals for your detox programme include buckwheat and millet. The whole grains of these cereals can be boiled like rice, or they can be bought as flakes or flour. Ask your local health food store which they stock.

Certain grains should not be included in a detox programme. The chief amongst these is wheat, which contains gluten, a sticky glue-like substance. A surprising number of people find gluten hard to digest and it causes them wind, indigestion and other digestive disturbances.

Wheat is one of the most common causes of food allergies, but it is used so widely – in bread, biscuits (cookies), cakes, breakfast cereals, pasta, noodles and many processed goods – that many sufferers remain quite unaware that they are sensitive to it. Try to avoid wheat altogether while you are following a detox programme. You may find this quite tricky at first, especially if you enjoy bread. Remember, however, you can use rice cakes for sandwiches. Many health food stores and supermarkets now stock gluten-free bread and you can eat small quantities of this or, better still, use the recipe on page 186 to make a Detox Loaf. This is especially good toasted. You can also find gluten-free pasta and noodles on the supermarket shelf.

Rye, barley and oats also contain gluten, so it is a good idea to avoid these while you detox.

Pulses, nuts and seeds

Pulses, nuts and seeds provide protein, as well as fibre, vitamins and minerals for your detox diet. Supermarkets sell a wonderful range of interesting dried beans and pulses these days – from kidney beans to chick peas (garbanzos) and different kinds of lentils. Buy fresh packets of dried beans to cook while you are detoxing, rather than resurrecting ancient packages from the depths of your cupboard.

Dried beans and pulses (except orange lentils) need soaking before they are cooked. All dried beans need thorough cooking, starting with a rapid boil for about 15 minutes. Never eat them raw. An excellent way to speed up the cooking of dried beans and pulses is to pop a strip of dried kombu seaweed into the pan. This helps to tenderise the beans and make them more digestible. Seaweed is also extremely good for you and a perfect detox food. You will find kombu in health food stores.

You can use cans of beans in an absolute emergency, but make sure you are not buying varieties cooked in sauce. Drain them extremely thoroughly, then rinse off any remaining salty water before you use them

All kinds of nuts are good for your detox diet, with the exception of peanuts. These in fact are not nuts at all, but belong to the pea family and are usually avoided during detoxing because they can be inclined to develop microscopic moulds.

All nuts should be bought as fresh as possible, and unblanched if available, so you get the benefit of the fibre in the skins. Never buy salted or roasted nuts or nuts with flavoured coatings. Just before you use the nuts, gently toast them for a minute or two under the grill (broiler) or in a dry pan to bring out their flavour. Sunflower, pumpkin and sesame seeds are also tasty, nutritious additions to your detox diet and make excellent snacks.

Bean and seed sprouts are amongst the very best foods you can eat while you detox. They are easy to digest and packed with protein, vitamins and minerals. You will find moong bean sprouts in the chiller cabinet of most supermarkets, and many health food stores sell the tasty cress-like shoots of sprouted alfalfa seeds. Mustard, cress, and other growing salads are also sprouts, of course, and extremely good for you.

It is very easy to grow your own bean and seed sprouts. Little green moong beans, alfalfa seeds and sesame seeds, for example, are all available from health food stores and are suitable for sprouting. Simply soak about one tablespoonful for about half an hour in water, then place them in a bowl or jar and rinse daily until they start to sprout. Pick out and discard any that go soggy or discoloured. Moong beans do best in the dark with a weight on them – perhaps a weighted plate.

Oils
Good-quality oils are important in your detox programme. Buy best-quality, organic and cold-pressed if possible. Do not use ordinary cooking oil and never reheat any kind of oil – clean the pan and start again with fresh oil each time.

Cold-pressed extra virgin olive oil is the best variety to use every day and especially for cooking. Other useful kinds include richly flavoured walnut oil which is delicious in salad dressings and dips, sesame oil which has a warm nutty taste and is especially good for stir-fries, and sweet almond oil which is ideal for sweet dishes.

Fish, tofu and chicken
Fish is one of the best protein foods you can eat when you are on a detox programme – try to include it in your diet at least once every other day. White fish such as cod, haddock, hake, halibut, plaice, coley and pollack are easily digested and a good source of protein and vitamins. Oil-rich fish such as trout, salmon, herring, mackerel, pilchards and sprats have the bonus of providing valuable fish oils.

In an emergency you can use canned fish, but make sure it is not in a sauce, and do drain it thoroughly before use. Smoked fish should be eaten only very occasionally and in moderation.

Tofu is bean curd made from soya beans; it is a traditional food from Japan where it is widely eaten. You can buy it in a solid block or in semi-liquid form from supermarkets and health food stores. It is an excellent low-fat form of protein, and although it does not really taste of anything, it readily absorbs the flavours of any marinade – lemon juice, soy sauce, garlic, finely chopped onions or herbs for example. It can be used in stir-fries, dips and as a tasty non-dairy alternative to cheese (see page 98). Try to buy organic tofu.

If you are a meat eater, you can have chicken or turkey while you are on a detox diet, but try not to eat it more than three times a week. Always buy the best quality you can afford, ideally organic or at least free-range and corn-fed, and trim off any fat before you cook it. Try to eat only small portions while you are detoxing. Do not eat goose or duck as these are too fatty.

Dairy and non-dairy produce
You should avoid cows'-milk products – milk, cheese, butter and yoghurt – while you are detoxing. A surprising number of people find cows' milk difficult to digest; many

find they are slightly allergic to it and that it creates excess mucus in their sinuses.

Sheep's milk and goats' milk are not as difficult to digest and many folk who cannot tolerate cows' milk find they can cope with these. Look out for goats' cheese, sheep's cheeses such as Feta (don't eat too much, because it is very salty), and goats' and sheep's yoghurt.

Soya milk, now widely available from supermarkets, is a useful alternative to dairy milk. You can buy it slightly sweetened with apple juice if you like, but try to get an organic variety if possible. You can also buy soya yoghurt (or make your own, see page 171). Other useful kinds of non-dairy milk include almond milk and rice milk. Make sure they do not have added sugar or artificial ingredients.

Herbs, spices and flavourings

Don't sprinkle salt over your food while you are following a detox programme, and try to keep salt in cooking to an absolute minimum. Try using a good sea salt or herb salt, and add it sparingly at the end of cooking after tasting carefully. Never add salt to vegetables during cooking.

Lemon juice, cider vinegar, balsamic vinegar, herbs and spices can all be used to add piquancy to a dish and minimise the amount of salt you need. You can also use good-quality Japanese soy sauce, but make sure the brand you buy does not contain additives such as sugar, caramel, or wheat. Tamari soy sauce is a traditional variety of Japanese soy sauce which is additive-free and gives a rich, savoury flavour to dishes. It is expensive, but you will only need to use small quantities.

You can use lots of fresh herbs in your cooking, and in salads. Several kinds are considered to be especially good for detoxing, including:
- **Parsley,** reputed to be a great kidney tonic
- **Fennel** and **dill,** to aid digestion
- **Mint,** to help digestion
- **Rosemary,** antiseptic and cleansing
- **Coriander** (cilantro), to assist digestion

Spices are also considered useful for detoxing, especially ground ginger and chilli powder; and coriander, dill (dill weed), caraway and fennel seeds will all help digestion.

Try adding these to recipes which include beans, cabbage or other foods that you find difficult to digest.

Supplements
You will find a range of different health supplements in your health food store, as well as vitamins and minerals. Some supplements, such as those listed below, are specifically intended to help detoxing.
- **Psyllium** and **linseed** add fibre to your diet and help flush through the system.
- **Milk thistle** has been used for centuries as a liver tonic.
- **Dandelion**, both the roots and leaves, have long been used as a tonic. You can pick your own young leaves to add to salads.
- **Aloe vera** helps digestion and promotes good bacteria in the gut.

FOODS TO AVOID

While you are detoxing you should avoid:
- Processed foods or foods with artificial additives or added sugar
- White and brown sugar
- Cows' milk products including cheese, butter and yoghurt
- Wheat and foods made with wheat, such as bread, cakes, pasta, noodles, biscuits
- Rye, barley and oats
- Tea and coffee
- Chocolate
- Eggs
- Red meat
- Margarines, other hard fats and cheap cooking oils
- Ketchup (catsup) and other bottled and prepared sauces
- Alcohol
- Fizzy soft drinks, squashes and cordials

Some detox nutritionists also advise omitting tomatoes and spinach from a detox diet, because of their oxalic acid content, and mushrooms and dried fruit because of the tiny yeasts that may be living on them.

PREPARATION AND COOKING

Preparation and cooking for a detox diet can be as simple as you want it to be. But there are some basic principles you should follow.

- Do not prepare food in advance; that way it is eaten as fresh as possible.
- Do not soak fresh vegetables in water before cooking.
- Cook vegetables until they are only just done, no more.
- Steam rather than boil.
- Drain vegetables immediately they are cooked.
- Do not keep leftovers for more than one day.
- Do not peel organic fruit and vegetables unless absolutely necessary.
- Add seasoning at the end of cooking to avoid over-salting.

WHAT ELSE TO DO

While you are following the detox diet, you should be making some gentle changes to other aspects of your life. These changes will help to make you feel fitter, healthier and more relaxed.

Exercise

Exercise helps the digestive system work properly. It is also a great stress releaser. If you are not getting enough exercise during the week, you probably feel sluggish and lacking in energy. You may also be constipated.

While you detox you should aim to do at least 20 minutes' exercise every day.

If you are very unfit, or totally exhausted when you start the detox programme, you should start exercising very gently indeed. Begin, perhaps with a gentle 20-minute walk after dinner each evening.

Once you are feeling more energetic, you can then move on to perhaps swimming twice a week, cycling at the weekend, regular visits to the gym, exercise classes or even walking briskly to and from work. Vigorous digging in the garden is excellent exercise, as are hill walking and dancing.

Rest

Proper rest is an essential part of the detox programme. If you have trouble getting to sleep at night, try gentle exercise to help you relax, then take a warm bath. Some herb teas are especially good for relaxation before bedtime. Look at the range available in your health food store or supermarket.

Most people need a short rest in the middle of the day. Many of us feel sleepy after lunch, for example, but find it hard to take time out to relax briefly, digest our meal and recharge our batteries. You should give yourself a proper break at midday – that way you will find you are much more efficient during the afternoon; try to organise your day to allow for this. Even if you are eating your midday meal at your office desk, make sure you lay aside your work for half an hour. Read the newspaper or a few pages of a novel, or go and sit in the park for 20 minutes. Don't just keep working through regardless.

Relaxation

There are lots of ways you can help yourself relax. You could try meditation. There are various well-established and effective meditation techniques, so find a book on the subject, or go to a meditation teacher.

You could also learn some simple yoga exercises, which not only stretch and tone the body, but also help develop useful breathing and relaxation techniques. Again, there are lots of self-help books on yoga for beginners, as well as local classes in many areas.

Aromatherapy has become tremendously popular in recent years. You could treat yourself to a session with a trained aromatherapist, or simply buy some relaxing aromatherapy oils and enjoy a warm, scented bath. However, do not use essential oils if you are pregnant or have sensitive skin, without first consulting a trained aromatherapist. Pure essential oils should never be applied directly to your skin.

Massage is another wonderful way of relaxing tense and tired muscles and relieving aches and pains. You could book yourself a session with a trained masseur, or use a self-help book to guide you through some simple massage techniques you can use yourself.

How long should a detox programme last? A weekend, a week, a month?

A one-week programme certainly gives your system a good chance to start working efficiently again and you should begin to feel the benefits of good-quality food, well-balanced nutrition and a more efficient digestive system. Indeed, even a weekend detox will leave you feeling healthier. But if you really want long-term benefits, you need to carry on the good habits for longer than two to seven days. Try keeping to the detox programme for a month, then you will start reaping solid benefits.

For the first week, you can simply follow the recommended seven-day eating plan on pages 30–36. After that, you will be well into the swing of things and be able to choose from the 90-odd recipes in this book to plan your own interesting and varied eating programme, adapting the recipes to suit your own tastes and preferences.

And by the time you have finished your detox programme, you will, hopefully, have developed a real taste for good food and healthy eating, and learned habits that will stay with you and help to keep you feeling fit, energetic and healthy, maintaining your system at peak efficiency.

NOTES ON THE RECIPES

- Do not mix metric, imperial and American measures. Follow one set only.
- American terms are given in brackets.
- All spoon measures are level: 1 tsp = 5ml; 1 tbsp = 15ml
- Use organic produce wherever possible. All fruit and vegetables should be washed, cored and seeded where necessary before use. There is no need to peel or scrape organic root vegetables such as carrots and potatoes but non-organic produce should have the skins removed in the usual way. Sweet potatoes and yams should also be peeled, as there have been recent reports of high levels of chemicals found on some supermarket yams.
- Ensure that all produce is as fresh as possible and in good condition.
- Always use fresh herbs unless dried are specifically called for. If it is necessary to use dried herbs, use half the quantity stated. Chopped frozen varieties are much better than dried. There is no substitute for fresh parsley and coriander (cilantro).
- Always preheat the oven unless you are using a fan-assisted one and cook on the centre shelf, unless otherwise stated.

7-DAY MENU PLAN

The following seven-day eating plan is based on seven simple daily rules. Once you are familiar with these rules, you can use them to plan your own day's eating from the recipes in the book. Each day, make sure you have:

- 1.75 litres/3 pints fluid
- At least three meals
- At least two raw food dishes
- Three servings of fruit
- At least two servings of vegetables or salad
- Two servings of grain
- Two servings from: fish, beans or pulses, tofu, chicken, nuts and seeds, or non-dairy produce

On pages 30–36 you will find seven days of menus. These will give you an idea of how you can put together a tasty, varied and balanced day's eating from the detox recipes in the book. Do remember that this eating plan is not a slimming diet. You should eat enough of the suggested foods in the menus to feel satisfied and if you become hungry between meals you should have an extra snack.

There may be some days, of course, when you really don't have the time or energy to make all the dishes suggested. In which case, here are some ideas for speedy, healthy alternatives that you can use to fill yourself up.

Quick breakfasts
Fresh fruit shake: use a blender to whiz a banana with a generous mugful of soya or goats' milk, some almonds and a little honey. Make sure the nuts are fully blended.

Fast lunches
Cheese and rice cakes: top rice cakes with goats' cheese, Feta or other cheese not made with cows' milk. Add some or all of the following: sliced apple, onion, cress, olives, avocado, grapes. Eat with fresh fruit and a handful of mixed nuts and seeds.
Tuna and rice cakes: use canned tuna, well drained, to top rice cakes, along with some or all of the following: lettuce, sliced apple, olives, grapes, watercress, onion,

chopped baby sweetcorn (corn), Detox Mayonnaise (see page 91). Eat with fresh fruit and a handful or two of mixed nuts and seeds.

Simple suppers

Corn and salmon: steam or boil corn cobs and serve with a can of red salmon, Detox Mayonnaise (see page 91) or Mustard Dressing (see page 102), plus rice cakes or slices of Detox Loaf (see page 186) and plenty of green salad.

Fish, rice and peas: allow about 50 g/2 oz/½ cup round wholegrain rice per person. Cook, then mix with a well drained can of kidney beans and a can of tuna or salmon. Roughly chop some raw vegetables and fruit – whatever you have to hand: carrots, cucumber, apple, spring onions (scallions), (bell) pepper, garlic, pineapple – and mix it in.

Jacket potato: microwave or oven-bake one large jacket potato per person, then fill with one of the following: goats' cheese, Feta, well drained canned fish, or well drained canned beans tossed in Detox Mayonnaise (see page 91). Serve with lots of green salad leaves.

Easy desserts

Fruit and yoghurt: chop bananas, apples, orange, fresh dates, figs or other fruit into sheep's, goats' or soya yoghurt. Stir in a drizzle of honey or pure maple syrup if liked.

Fruit compôte: stew a large cooking (tart) apple or other fruit with fresh, chopped dates in orange juice. Serve with yoghurt.

Speedy snacks

Popcorn: follow instructions on the packet, cooking in olive oil rather than butter; do not add butter or sugar; simply sprinkle with a little herb salt, if liked, before eating hot or cold. Store in an airtight container.

Mixed nuts: mix together your favourite shelled nuts and seeds. Store in airtight container if not using immediately.

Fruit: fresh fruit including avocados, dates, figs, bananas, grapes, apples and pears.

Olives: any kind, well rinsed to remove excess salt.

DAY ONE

On waking   Hot water or wake-up drink of your
choice (see pages 38–9)

Breakfast   Fresh fruit juice of your choice
(see pages 53–7)
Mixed Grain Porridge (see page 51),
drizzled with honey or maple syrup
Hot toasted Detox Loaf (see page 186),
spread with Almond and Apricot
Topping (see page 185)
Herbal tea, if liked

Mid-morning   Herbal tea, fresh juice or mineral water
1 handful of Savoury Sunflower Seeds
(see page 87) or mixed nuts

Lunch   1 generous portion of Vegetable Salad
with Leeks, Celeriac and Broad Beans
(see page 104)
Rice cakes topped with Olive, Sweet
Pepper and Nut Pâté (see page 82) or
Feta cheese and salad leaves
1 or 2 fresh fruits of your choice
Mineral water

Teatime   Herbal tea or Clear Vegetable Stock
(see page 15)
Fresh fruit such as banana, figs or dates, if
you are hungry

Supper   Parsnip and Coriander Soup (see page 59)
Trout Fillets with Beetroot, Orange and
Fennel Sauce (see page 121)
Mixed Green Salad (see page 89) and
Savoury Vegetable Rice (see page 162)
Luxury Fruit Salad (see page 180), served
with Creamy Vanilla Sauce (see
page 181) or Home-made Yoghurt
(see page 171), or 1 or 2 fresh fruits

Bedtime   Hot water or herbal tea

DAY TWO

On waking   Hot water or wake-up drink of your
           choice (see pages 38–9)

Breakfast   Herbal tea and/or fresh juice of your
           choice (see pages 53–7)
           Papaya and Citrus Platter (see page 41)
           Galettes Stuffed with Tuna and Sweetcorn
           (see page 46)

Mid-morning   Herbal tea, fresh juice or mineral water
           1–2 handfuls of fresh dates or Savoury
           Sunflower Seeds (see page 87)

Lunch   Aubergine and Goats' Cheese Pâté
           (see page 86), spread on rice cakes or
           thin slices of Detox Loaf (see page 186)
           1 generous portion of California Salad
           with Citrus Dressing (see page 92)
           1 or 2 fresh fruits of your choice
           Mineral water, herbal tea or fresh fruit
           juice

Teatime   Herbal tea or Clear Vegetable Stock
           (see page 15)
           Fresh fruit such as avocado, dates, figs, or
           banana, if you are hungry

Supper   Beetroot and Pear Salad (see page 99)
           Chinese Lemon Chicken (see page 140),
           served with rice and Speedy Stir-fried
           Vegetables (see page 164)
           Fresh Peach and Maple Syrup Sorbet
           (see page 179), served with Almond
           and Rice Fingers (see page 183)
           Mineral water

Bedtime   Herbal tea or hot water

DAY THREE

On waking   Hot water or wake-up drink of your choice (see pages 38–9)

Breakfast   Herbal tea and/or fresh juice of your choice (see pages 53–7)
Toasted Grapefruit, Pineapple and Almonds (see page 42)
Nutty Muesli (see page 45), topped with Home-made Yoghurt (see page 171) and fruit

Mid-morning   Herbal tea, fresh juice or mineral water
1 banana or 1 handful of fresh dates

Lunch   Rice cakes topped with goats' cheese or Tofu Cheese (see page 98) and alfalfa sprouts plus 1 generous portion of Mediterranean Mixed Bean Salad (see page 108)
1 or 2 fresh fruits of your choice
Herbal tea, mineral water or fresh fruit juice

Teatime   Herbal tea or Clear Vegetable Stock (see page 15)
Fresh fruit such as banana, figs or dates or a handful of nuts, if you are hungry

Supper   Chilled Watercress and Avocado Soup (see page 63)
Mediterranean Fishcakes with Chargrilled Vegetables (see page 124)
Olive Oil Mash with Wilted Rocket Leaves (see page 154)
Mixed Green Salad (see page 89)
Cinnamon Rice Pudding (see page 175) with stewed or fresh fruit of your choice

Bedtime   Herbal tea or hot water

DAY FOUR

On waking   Hot water or wake-up drink of your
               choice (see pages 38–9)

Breakfast   Herbal tea and/or fresh juice of your
               choice (see pages 53–7)
               Pineapple Blush (see page 43)
               Crispy Vegetable Patties
               (see page 48)

Mid-morning Herbal tea, fresh juice or mineral water
               1 handful of grapes, fresh dates or your
               favourite mixed nuts

Lunch   Corn Chowder (see page 62) with rice
               cakes or fingers of hot toasted Detox
               Loaf (see page 186)
               1 portion of Celery, Apple and Mixed Nut
               Salad (see page 116)
               1 or 2 fresh fruits of your choice
               Mineral water

Teatime   Herbal tea or Clear Vegetable Stock
               (see page 15)
               Fresh fruit such as dates, figs or banana, if
               you are hungry

Supper   Mixed Melon Starter (see page 70)
               Tuna Steak in a Hazelnut and Herb Crust
               (see page 120)
               Savoury Vegetable Rice (see page 162) or
               plain rice, if liked, and Mixed Green
               Salad (see page 89)
               Harlequin Poached Pears (see page 176)
               with Home-made Yoghurt (see page
               171) or Creamy Vanilla Sauce
               (see page 181), or 1 or 2 fresh fruits of
               your choice

Bedtime   Herbal tea or hot water

DAY FIVE

On waking	Hot water or wake-up drink of your choice (see pages 38–9)
Breakfast	Herbal tea or fresh juice of your choice (see pages 53–7) Fresh or stewed fruit of your choice Welsh Breakfast (see page 50)
Mid-morning	Herbal tea, fresh juice or mineral water 1–2 handfuls of Savoury Sunflower Seeds (see page 87), well rinsed olives, or your favourite mixed nuts
Lunch	Crudités with Creamy Tofu Dip (see page 78) and rice cakes, if liked 1 generous portion of Potato and Celery Salad (see page 114), sprinkled with a handful of walnuts 1 or 2 fresh fruits of your choice Mineral water or herbal tea, or Clear Vegetable Stock (see page 15)
Teatime	Herbal tea or Clear Vegetable Stock (see page 15) Fresh fruit or popcorn (see page 29), if you are hungry
Supper	Asparagus with Tahini Dressing (see page 73) Monkfish Stir-fry (see page 122) Fragrant Rice Salad (see page 106) or plain rice, if liked, with a large Mixed Green Salad (see page 89) Spiced Baked Bananas (see page 173)
Bedtime	Herbal tea or hot water

DAY SIX

On waking	Hot water or wake-up drink of your choice (see pages 38–9)
Breakfast	Herbal tea or fresh juice of your choice (see pages 53–7) 1 generous portion of Fruit Bowl (see page 44) Tofu Scramble (see page 85), served hot and piled on crisply toasted Detox Loaf (see page 186)
Mid-morning	Herbal tea, fresh juice or mineral water Fresh fruit such as dates, figs or banana, or 1–2 handfuls of popcorn (see page 29)
Lunch	Hazelnut and Lemon Butter (see page 79), spread on rice cakes and topped with fresh growing salad such as mustard and cress or alfalfa sprouts 1 generous portion of Feta, Olive and Summer Herb Salad (see page 96) 1 or 2 fresh fruits of your choice Mineral water or herbal tea, or cup of Clear Vegetable Stock (see page 15)
Teatime	Herbal tea or Clear Vegetable Stock (see page 15) 1–2 handfuls of Savoury Sunflower Seeds (see page 87), if you are hungry
Supper	Carrot and Coriander Soup (see page 59) Paella (see page 142), served with a large Mixed Green Salad (see page 89) Carob-coated Pears (see page 182)
Bedtime	Herbal tea or hot water

DAY SEVEN

On waking   Hot water or wake-up drink of your
choice (see pages 38–9)

Breakfast   Rice Porridge (see page 51), drizzled with
honey and served with fresh fruit or
stewed apricots
Hot Crisp Savoury Toasts (see page 84)
Herbal tea or fresh juice of your choice
(see pages 53–7)

Mid-morning   Herbal tea, fresh juice or mineral water
Fresh fruit such as dates, figs, banana,
apple or pear

Lunch   Hummus with Crudités (see page 80)
and rice cakes, if liked
1 generous portion of Rice and Cashew
Nut Salad with Lime Dressing
(see page 94)
1 or 2 fresh fruits of your choice
Mineral water or herbal tea, or cup of
Clear Vegetable Stock (see page 15)

Teatime   Herbal tea or Clear Vegetable Stock
(see page 15)
1–2 handfuls of popcorn (see page 29)
or Savoury Sunflower Seeds (see page
87), if you are hungry

Supper   Icelandic Beetroot and Haddock Salad
(see page 100)
Speedy Stir-fried Vegetables (see page 164),
served with a large Mixed Green Salad
(see page 89)
Summer Fruits Crumble (see page 178),
served with Home-made Yoghurt
(see page 171) or Creamy Vanilla
Sauce (see page 181)

Bedtime   Herbal tea or hot water

EARLY MORNING WAKE-UP DRINKS

Forget those cups of tea or coffee –
they're off-limits when you're on a
detox diet. The drinks on the following
pages will do a far better job of getting
rid of that muzzy early-morning feeling
and give your day a really healthy start.

Lemon Zester

Lemon juice is considered to be one of the best liver tonics. Use organic lemons if you can, and add thin strips of lemon zest to the water. Twist the strips first to release the lemon oil, which has beneficial anti-fungal properties. Do not use zest from waxed lemons. This drink is also refreshing drunk cold at other times of the day.

SERVES 2

450 ml/¾ pt/2½ cups boiling water

1 lemon

1 Pour the boiling water into a jug. If you are using an organic lemon, wipe it, then carefully peel three or four thin strips of zest from the fruit.

2 Twist the strips of zest to release the oils, then submerge them in the boiling water.

3 Squeeze the juice from the lemon and stir into the water.

4 Leave for about 5 minutes before pouring into individual glasses.

Ginger and Lime Wake-up

Ginger has excellent digestion-calming properties, so if your system wakes up in the morning a little out of sorts, this is the drink for you. Juice from a ripe lime is gentler than lemon, though you can use lemon if you prefer.

SERVES 2

---

450 ml/¾ pt/2½ cups boiling water

....

Freshly squeezed juice of 1 ripe lime

....

3 cm/1¼ in piece of fresh root ginger, peeled

....

1 Pour the water into a jug and stir in the lime juice.

2 Crush the ginger in a garlic press, allowing the juice to fall into the hot water.

3 Remove the crushed root from the garlic press and stir it into the hot water. Allow it to stand for about 4 minutes.

4 Strain into two glasses.

Cider Vinegar Starter

Cider vinegar is widely valued as an all-round tonic for the digestion, with useful anti-bacterial properties too. However, it is quite powerful, so if your digestion is delicate, choose Ginger and Lime Wake-up (see above).

SERVES 2

---

450 ml/¾ pt/2½ cups boiling water

....

30 ml/2 tbsp cider vinegar

....

1 Pour the boiling water into a jug. Leave for a few moments to cool slightly.

2 Stir in the cider vinegar, then pour into two glasses.

BREAKFASTS

Breakfast, it is often said, is the most important meal of the day and while you are detoxing you should make sure you allow time for this meal. In this section there is something for every taste, whether you like your breakfast fresh and fruity, warm and filling or really hearty and satisfying.

Papaya and Citrus Platter

Papayas are excellent detox foods, rich in useful digestive enzymes. You can simply slice the fruit, remove the pips and scoop the succulent pinkish-orange flesh straight out of the skin, as you do with avocados, but I like my papaya peeled and thinly sliced first, fanned out prettily on a plate and sprinkled with lemon and lime juice.

SERVES 2

1 papaya

½ lemon, cut into wedges

½ lime, cut into wedges

1 Cut the papaya in half and scoop out the seeds and stray fibres from the centre of each half.

2 Carefully peel the fruit and cut each half into about eight slices.

3 Arrange the slices on individual plates in a fan shape.

4 Serve on individual plates with lemon and lime wedges ready for squeezing over the fruit.

Toasted Grapefruit and Pineapple with Almonds

The grapefruit should be heated, but not cooked. Use pink grapefruit rather than the acidic yellow variety and you will probably not need extra sweetening. If you do, add a little drizzle of mild runny honey before toasting. For a change, try toasted grapefruit and halved bananas, or toasted halved banana with slices of peach.

SERVES 2

---

1 pink grapefruit

....

4 slices of fresh pineapple, trimmed, halved and any core removed

....

10 ml/2 tsp sweet almond oil

....

20–25 g/¾–1 oz flaked (slivered) almonds

....

1 Preheat the grill (broiler) to medium. Slice the grapefruit in two and use a sharp knife to score around each half, to separate the flesh from the peel. Be careful not to puncture the peel. Then slice three-quarters of the way down between the segments, to help loosen them.

2 Using a pastry brush, brush the tops of the grapefruit halves and the pineapple slices with almond oil.

3 Place the grapefruit and pineapple on a grill pan and grill (broil) for 2–3 minutes.

4 Add the almond flakes to the side of the grill pan and return to the heat for about 1 minute until the almond flakes begin to colour. Watch them carefully and do not let them turn more than the palest brown.

5 Remove the pan from the heat and arrange the grapefruit and pineapple on individual dishes, then sprinkle over the toasted almond flakes. Serve immediately.

Pineapple Blush

This delicately pink fruit cream makes an excellent breakfast dish, or a refreshing light dessert. A well ripened pineapple will provide enough sweetness for most tastes but if you need more add about 5 ml/1 tsp organic clear honey to the blender mix, or pure sugar-free fruit juice concentrate (available from health food stores).

SERVES 4

9 ripe strawberries

1 small sweet pineapple, peeled and cut into cubes

200 g/7 oz/scant 1 cup tofu or live sheep's, goats' or soya yoghurt

1 Hull the strawberries and set aside four evenly shaped fruit for decoration.

2 Place the remaining strawberries with the pineapple and tofu or yoghurt in blender.

3 Blend for about 30 seconds until the mixture is smooth and frothy.

4 Pour into glass dishes and refrigerate for about 1 hour until chilled.

5 Decorate with the remaining strawberries, halved or sliced, and serve immediately.

Fruit Bowl

You can use any fruit you like for this, but banana and dates are especially satisfying. Use organic unsulphured apricots if you can (available from health food stores); they're not only better for you, but also have a gorgeous brown-sugar-cum-toffee flavour.

SERVES 2

---

6 dried apricots

....

75 g/3 oz/generous ¾ cup rice or millet flakes

....

300 ml/½ pt/1¼ cups fresh apple juice, orange juice or non-dairy milk

....

2 ripe bananas, peeled and chopped

....

2 small sweet apples, cored and chopped

....

6–8 fresh dates, stoned (pitted) and roughly chopped

....

Goats', sheep's or soya yoghurt (optional)

....

1 If you like your apricots presoaked, place in a bowl, cover with water and leave in a cool place overnight. Drain, chop and divide between two individual dishes.

2 Divide the rice or millet flakes between the two dishes and pour half the juice or milk into each dish. Leave to soak for about 15 minutes.

3 Divide the fruit between the two dishes. Serve, with yoghurt, if liked.

Nutty Muesli

This breakfast is guaranteed to sustain you through till mid-morning. Add any chopped raw fruit you like. I do not usually weigh these ingredients out, but simply add about one spoonful of each kind of nut to three spoonfuls of rice or millet flakes. The quantities don't have to be exact.

SERVES 2

90 ml/6 tbsp/generous ¾ cup rice or millet flakes

300 ml/½ pt/1¼ cups fresh apple juice, orange juice or non-dairy milk

25 g/1 oz/¼ cup whole unblanched almonds

25 g/1 oz/¼ cup whole hazelnuts (filberts)

25 g/1 oz/¼ cup sunflower seeds

25 g/1 oz/¼ cup pumpkin seeds

1 ripe banana and/or other fruit, such as an apple or pear, if liked

Goats', sheep's or soya yoghurt (optional)

1 Place the rice or millet flakes in a medium bowl and pour the juice or milk over them. Leave to stand for about 15 minutes.

2 Add the nuts and seeds and mix the ingredients together.

3 Divide between two individual dishes. Slice the bananas (and other fruit, if liked) over the top, add a dollop of yoghurt and serve.

Galettes Stuffed with Tuna and Sweetcorn

These traditional French pancakes, made with buckwheat flour, are stuffed with fresh tuna and sweetcorn (corn) for a delicious savoury breakfast, while generous quantities of fresh parsley and lemon juice help to make this a great detox dish. Serve the galettes with slices of leftover potato browned under the grill (broiler) for a really substantial breakfast. Low-sodium baking powder and specialist flours are available from health food stores.

SERVES 4
550 g/1¼ lb fresh tuna steak
Freshly squeezed juice of 1 lemon, plus extra for sprinkling
25 ml/1½ tbsp tamari soy sauce
60 ml/4 tbsp cold-pressed extra virgin olive oil, plus extra for frying (sautéing)
100 g/4 oz/1 cup buckwheat flour
50 g/2 oz/½ cup potato flour
10 ml/2 tsp low-sodium baking powder
250 ml/8 fl oz/1 cup soya milk
200 ml/7 fl oz/scant 1 cup water
2 sweetcorn (corn) cobs
45 ml/3 tbsp chopped flatleaf parsley
8 small sprigs of parsley, to garnish

1 Place the tuna in a shallow non-metallic dish. Mix together the lemon juice, soy sauce and 15 ml/1 tbsp olive oil and pour over the tuna. Leave to marinate in a cool place for at least 30 minutes (overnight in a fridge is ideal).

2 To make the pancake batter, put the flours and baking powder in a large mixing bowl. Gradually whisk in the milk, the water and the oil, then whisk for a further 30 seconds. Leave to stand while you cook the filling.

3 Bring a large pan of water to the boil, add the sweetcorn and boil for 7–8 minutes, until tender. Drain, then strip the cobs of their kernels by cutting down the length of the heads with a stout knife.

4 Remove the tuna from the marinade and place on a grill (broiler) pan, then pour the marinade over the fish. Cook under a medium, preheated grill for about 3 minutes, then turn and cook on the other side, basting and checking very carefully that it does not dry out or overcook.

5 Remove from the grill as soon as it is cooked. Cut into 1 cm/½ in thick strips, place in a warmed dish with the cooking juices, add the sweetcorn and gently stir to combine the ingredients. Cover and set aside.

6 Now make the pancakes. Heat a small amount of oil (less than 5 ml/1 tsp) in an omelette pan. Swirl it or wipe it around the pan to coat the surface.

7 Whisk the batter mixture again for about 10 seconds, then carefully pour 45–60 ml/3–4 tbsp of batter into the pan, tilting the pan so that the batter covers the base evenly.

8 Cook the pancake for about 1 minute, then turn it over and cook the other side.

9 When cooked, spoon about 15 ml/1 tbsp of the tuna and sweetcorn mixture over one half of the pancake, sprinkle with parsley and a few drops of lemon juice, then fold the pancake over the filling. Remove from the pan and place on a heated roasting tray in the oven. Repeat with the remaining pancake batter and stuffing, to make eight galettes in all.

10 Serve garnished with sprigs of parsley.

Crispy Vegetable Patties

You can use leftover vegetables and rice for this simple tasty breakfast dish. Allow proportions of at least two-thirds vegetables to one-third rice to ensure the little cakes hold together when cooking. Starchy vegetables such as potato also help them cohere.

SERVES 2–4
350 g/12 oz cold cooked vegetables, such as potato, carrot, beans, peas, squash, courgettes (zucchini)
175 g/6 oz/1½ cups cold cooked wholegrain round rice
5 ml/1 tsp chopped parsley
5 ml/1 tsp chopped thyme
5 ml/1 tsp snipped chives
2.5 ml/½ tsp tamari soy sauce
2.5 ml/½ tsp freshly squeezed lemon juice
Freshly ground black pepper and a little sea salt
A pinch of cayenne (optional)
45 ml/3 tbsp rice or millet flakes or sesame seeds
5–10 ml/1–2 tsp potato or soya flour, if necessary
15 ml/1 tbsp olive oil
Sprigs of flatleaf parsley, to garnish

1 Make sure the vegetables are thoroughly drained. Vegetables with a high moisture content such as courgettes should be patted dry with kitchen paper (paper towels).

2 Place the vegetables in a large bowl and chop, then mash thoroughly with a potato masher or a fork. Do not use a blender as it will make the mixture too sticky.

3   Add the rice, herbs, soy sauce and lemon juice and mix thoroughly. Season with generous quantities of freshly ground black pepper, a little sea salt and a small pinch of cayenne, if liked.

4   If using large rice flakes to coat the patties, you will first need to crush them a little. Whiz very briefly in a food processor, or place in a polythene bag and crush briefly with a rolling pin. Pour the rice flakes, millet flakes or sesame seeds on to a large plate.

5   Form four large or eight small balls from the vegetable and rice mixture. If the mixture is too wet, mix in the potato or soya flour. One at a time, roll them in the rice or millet flakes or sesame seeds, then flatten them slightly and transfer to another plate.

6   Cover the plate and leave to stand in a cool place for about 15 minutes.

7   Heat the oil in a large frying pan (skillet) and cook the patties for about 5 minutes on each side until piping hot inside and crisp outside.

8   Serve immediately garnished with sprigs of parsley.

Welsh Breakfast

These crisply fried little cakes, a traditional Welsh breakfast dish called laverbread, are made from puréed seaweed. Here, the laverbread is served with fillets of trout to make a substantial cooked meal. Seaweed is an excellent detox food. You can buy laver in its dried Japanese form, called nori, *from most independent health food stores and some supermarkets.*

SERVES 2

10 g/scant ½ oz dried Japanese laver (nori)

5 ml/1 tsp fresh lemon juice

Freshly ground black pepper

120 g/4 oz/1 cup millet flakes

30 ml/2 tbsp cold-pressed extra virgin olive oil

2–3 medium trout fillets

Sea salt

Lemon wedges and sprigs of parsley, to garnish

---

1 Tear up the dried laver and place it in a saucepan. Cover it with water, bring to the boil and simmer, stirring, until the laver sheet has disintegrated and has formed a smooth purée.

2 Place the laver in a sieve (strainer) and drain it thoroughly. It must not be wet. Transfer to a mixing bowl and add 2.5 ml/½ tsp lemon juice, some black pepper and about 25–30 g/1–1½ oz millet flakes. Stir to make a stiff purée, then set aside for about 20 minutes.

3 Form four to six little cakes from the laver mixture, then roll them in some of the remaining millet flakes.

4 Heat 15 ml/1 tbsp oil in a frying pan (skillet) and begin to fry (sauté) the laver cakes gently, turning to make sure they crisp evenly.

5   Meanwhile, sprinkle the remaining lemon juice over the trout fillets, season with black pepper and a little sea salt, then roll them in the remaining millet flakes.

6   Heat the remaining oil in a separate pan and fry the trout for about 3 minutes each side.

7   Serve immediately garnished with lemon wedges and sprigs of parsley.

&

Mixed Grain Porridge

Be careful to stir the porridge while it is cooking because soya milk burns easily. For a change, try serving it with a purée of stewed dried apricots or fresh dates instead of honey or maple syrup and milk. Alternatively, for Rice Porridge, omit the millet flakes and use double the quantity of rice flakes.

SERVES 2

---

450 ml/¾ pt/2 cups soya milk, plus extra for pouring

40 g/1½ oz/generous ⅓ cup rice flakes

40 g/1½ oz/generous ⅓ cup millet flakes

15–30 ml/1–2 tbsp mild organic honey or pure maple syrup (optional)

---

1   Pour the milk into a medium saucepan and heat gently.

2   Gradually stir in the rice and millet flakes and continue for about 4 minutes, stirring all the time.

3   Stir in a little more soya milk if the mixture becomes too stiff.

4   Serve hot with a jug of soya milk for pouring. You may also want to add a drizzle of honey or maple syrup as well, especially if using unsweetened soya milk.

JUICES

Fresh juices are excellent for detoxing; they are highly cleansing, packed with nutrients, yet easy to digest. They can be drunk at any time of day and whether you want a cooling, thirst-quencher or a refreshing appetite-tingling starter, the recipes on the following pages are all delicious, healthy and simple to make.
Always buy organic produce for juices and use the freshest possible ingredients – squeeze your own orange, lemon and lime juices and buy other fresh juices from the chiller cabinet of your supermarket. If you are lucky enough to own a juicer then you can produce really wonderful juices, using every bit of the fruit. As a rough guide, two eating (dessert) apples should give around 175 ml/6 fl oz/¾ cup juice, and two medium oranges will yield around 200 ml/7 fl oz/1 cup juice. Make sure you use home-made juices immediately or they will discolour and lose their flavour and nutrients.

Mango, Apple and Ginger Kick-start

A marvellously cleansing breakfast drink to kick-start your morning, or to drink as a mid-morning refresher. Adjust the quantity of ginger you use according to taste; serve either thick and frothy or mixed with mineral water to make a longer drink.

SERVES 2

---

1 ripe mango

....

1 large eating (dessert) apple, chopped

....

5 mm/¼ in piece of fresh root ginger, peeled

....

1 Thinly peel the mango, taking care to lose as little flesh as possible. Cut the flesh away from the mango's flat central stone (pit), and chop into 2 cm/¾ in pieces. Scrape the stone to remove any remaining flesh – it can all be used.

2 Place the mango, apple and ginger in a blender and blend for about 30 seconds, or feed them into a juicer.

3 If using a blender, strain the liquid through a sieve (strainer), if liked, or serve thick and frothy.

Melon and Grape

This juice is as sweet and fragrant as nectar. Chill the fruit before juicing to make an exquisite ice-cold drink for warm summer afternoons. If you have an especially delicate digestion, you may find melon is indigestible when mixed with other fruits. If this is the case, drink melon juice by itself, and save your grapes for mixing with pineapple or papaya.

SERVES 2

½ medium melon (any kind)

15 grapes

1 Scoop out the melon seeds and discard, then remove the flesh from the rind. Cut into 2 cm/¾ in pieces.

2 Place the fruit in a blender and blend until smooth and frothy, or feed through a juicer.

3 If using a blender, strain the mixture through a sieve (strainer), if liked, before serving.

Melon and Banana

Sumptiously sweet, frothy and creamy, this is almost a dessert in its own right. Don't use a juicer for this – you will extract only a tiny drop of liquid from a single banana, so use a blender. Leave the melon in the fridge for a few hours before juicing if you want to drink this chilled, but don't refrigerate the banana. If your digestion is delicate, substitute very ripe peaches or pineapple for the melon in this recipe.

SERVES 2

½ ripe medium honeydew melon

1 large ripe banana

1. Scoop out the seeds from the melon, then cut the flesh from the peel and chop into 3 cm/1¼ in pieces.

2. Put the melon and banana pieces in a blender and blend for about 30 seconds until smooth and frothy.

Pink Citrus

Clementines or mandarins add a subtle flowery flavour to this pretty pink juice. Pink grapefruit are much less acidic than their yellow relatives, which have good flavour but generally need added sweetness.

SERVES 2

1 pink grapefruit

2–3 clementines or mandarins, depending on size

1. Peel the fruit, and remove any pips. Make sure almost all the white pith is removed from the grapefruit.

2. Break each fruit into chunks of 3–4 segments, then place in a blender and whiz for about 30 seconds until smooth and frothy. Alternatively, feed through a juicer.

3. If using a blender, strain before serving, if liked.

Grape and Papaya

Nothing could be more detoxing than combining these two excellent cleansers in a single glass of this creamy drink.

SERVES 2

---

1 papaya, quartered and seeded

225 g/8 oz seedless grapes

1 Place all the fruit in a blender and blend for about 20 seconds, until smooth and frothy. Alternatively, feed through a juicer.

2 If using a blender, strain through a sieve (strainer) before serving, if liked.

Beetroot and Mandarin

Raw beetroot (red beet) is considered by many detox nutritionists as the ultimate cleanser. Here, its sweet earthy flavour is complemented by the delicate acidity of citrus.

SERVES 2

---

1 medium beetroot, scrubbed and cut into 4 pieces

2 mandarins, peeled and pips removed

200 ml/7 fl oz/scant 1 cup water, if using a blender

1 Place the beetroot and mandarin in a blender with the water and blend for about 40 seconds until reduced to an almost-smooth consistency. Alternatively, feed through a juicer, omitting the water.

2 If using a blender, press firmly through a fine sieve (strainer).

Carrot, Orange and Mint

The orange and carrot in this glorious sunset-coloured juice combine to create an intriguing flavour. Scrape the carrots only if they are not organically grown. I like to use apple mint, or one of the other interesting varieties of mint which grow in my garden, but ordinary mint works just as well. Sip the juice through the sprigs of mint.

SERVES 2

1 medium orange, peeled and quartered

3 medium carrots, cut into chunks

2 sprigs of mint

1 Place the orange and carrot pieces in a blender, whiz for about 30 seconds until smooth and frothy, then strain, if liked. Alternatively, use a juicer.

2 Serve with a sprig of mint in each glass.

Cucumber and Grape

In this recipe, the grapes help to add sweetness to the juice, while removing the skin of the cucumber helps to prevent it being bitter.

SERVES 2

100 g/4 oz cucumber, peeled and cut into chunks

75 g/3 oz sweet white seedless grapes

Place the cucumber and grapes in a blender and whiz for about 20 seconds, then strain the juice through a fine sieve (strainer), if liked. Alternatively, use a juicer.

SOUPS

Soups are an ideal addition to a detox diet: they are quick and simple to prepare and you can include almost any fresh ingredients you like.
The best soups are made with fresh home-made stock (see page 15), but if you don't have any to hand or are in a hurry, boiling water plus an additive-free stock (boullion) cube, available from health food stores, will do.

Parsnip and Coriander Soup

Both coriander (cilantro) and chilli are useful additions to your detox diet. For a delicious change, replace the parsnips with the same weight of carrots, and add a 1 cm/½ in piece of ginger to the blender goblet in step 2.

SERVES 4

---

700 g/1½ lb parsnips, scrubbed and chopped

1 medium onion, peeled

1 bunch of fresh coriander

750 ml/1¼ pts/3 cups well flavoured vegetable stock

30 ml/ 2 tbsp freshly squeezed lemon juice

45 ml/3 tbsp fresh apple juice

½ small fresh chilli, seeded and chopped

Freshly ground black pepper

2 spring onions (scallions), finely chopped

---

1 Steam the parsnips and onion until only just tender.

2 When the parsnips and onion are cooked, leave to cool slightly before transferring to a blender goblet. Blend for about 50 seconds until smooth and creamy, then transfer to a large saucepan.

3 Wash the coriander, removing any roots and damaged leaves. Set aside a few leaves as garnish and roughly tear the rest.

4 Place the torn coriander in the blender with the stock, lemon and apple juices and the chopped chilli. Blend for about 30 seconds, then stir into the parsnip purée.

5 Reheat the soup, taking care not to allow it to boil, and season with freshly ground black pepper.

6 Serve garnished with finely chopped spring onion and coriander leaves.

Bortsch

This richly flavoured traditional Russian broth has a fabulous deep crimson-pink colour. Serve it with dramatic swirl of creamy white yoghurt and a piquant sprinkle of caraway seeds. If you can't get hold of raw beetroot (red beet), buy additive-free cooked whole beetroot – but not the kind that comes in vinegar.

SERVES 4

---

45 ml/3 tbsp cold-pressed extra virgin olive oil

2 onions, chopped

1 celery stick, chopped

1 medium carrot, chopped

150 g/5 oz cabbage, shredded

450 g/1 lb raw beetroot, scrubbed and trimmed

5 ml/1 tsp chopped rosemary

5 ml/1 tsp English mustard powder

800 ml/1⅓ pts/3½ cups well flavoured vegetable stock

Freshly ground black pepper

A few drops of freshly squeezed lemon juice

Sea salt, to taste

60 ml/4 tbsp goats', sheep's or soya yoghurt

1.5 ml/¼ tsp caraway seeds

1 Heat the oil in a large pan and fry (sauté) the onions, celery, carrot and cabbage in the oil. Grate the raw beetroot, then stir into the pan. Continue to cook the vegetables for 3–4 minutes until just softened but not browned.

2 If using cooked beetroot, slice fairly finely, and add to the pan now. Add the rosemary and mustard and continue to cook for about 3 minutes.

3 Add the stock to the pan, and simmer gently for a further 15–20 minutes. Season with plenty of freshly ground black pepper, a few drops of lemon juice and a little sea salt to taste.

4 Remove the pan from the heat and allow it to cool a little.

5 Place the mixture in a blender or, for a more textured soup, a food processor and whiz for about 30 seconds. You may have to process the mixture in batches.

6 Return to the saucepan and reheat. Pour into individual soup bowls. Swirl 15 ml/1 tbsp yoghurt on top of each bowl, then sprinkle on a few caraway seeds before serving immediately.

Corn Chowder

This substantial creamy soup makes an excellent supper or lunch dish served with a big green salad. If you like bread with your soup, make sure you use Detox Loaf (see page 186) rather than wheat bread.

SERVES 4

4 medium sweetcorn (corn) cobs

300 ml/½ pt/1¼ cups non-dairy milk (any kind, but rice milk works well)

30 ml/2 tbsp sesame oil

350 g/12 oz onions, sliced

400 g/14 oz potatoes, cut into 5 mm/¼ in dice

2.5 ml/½ tsp cider vinegar

Freshly ground black pepper

Sea salt, to taste

1 Boil the sweetcorn cobs in a large pan of water for about 10 minutes, or until the kernels are just tender. Drain the cobs and slice off the kernels cleanly with a sharp knife.

2 Place half the kernels in a blender with the milk. Blend to a medium-smooth purée.

3 Heat the oil in a large pan and fry (sauté) the onions until soft but not coloured.

4 Stir in the sweetcorn purée and potatoes and cook for about 5 minutes, until the potatoes are just tender.

5 Stir in the rest of the sweetcorn and the cider vinegar. Season with pepper and sea salt, to taste, and continue cooking for a further 2 minutes.

6 Serve in individual bowls with an extra grinding of black pepper over each.

Chilled Watercress and Avocado Soup

There are several versions of this soup – you can use good-quality clear stock, for example, instead of water, but I like the clean taste and simplicity of this version. The small rough-skinned avocados are better than the larger smooth-skinned variety because they have a richer, creamier flavour.

SERVES 4

About 900 ml/1½ pts/3¾ cups water

2 medium rough-skinned avocados

175 g/6 oz watercress

Freshly squeezed juice of 1 lemon

45 ml/3 tbsp mild creamy goats', sheep's or soya yoghurt

1 cm/½ in red chilli, seeded and chopped

Sea salt, to taste

A few thin strips of lemon zest, to garnish

---

1 About 2 hours before making the soup, place the water in a jug and refrigerate, along with all the other ingredients.

2 Peel and stone (pit) the avocados and place in a blender along with the watercress. Add the lemon juice, yoghurt and chilli and blend for about 20 seconds.

3 Gradually add enough of the the chilled water to make a consistency you like, blending the ingredients thoroughly.

4 Test for seasoning and add a little sea salt, if necessary.

5 Serve immediately in individual bowls, garnished with thin strips of lemon zest.

Thai Fish Soup

Any kind of white fish will do for this recipe – haddock, cod, coley or pollack. If at all possible you should use freshly grated coconut. If you can't get hold of a fresh coconut, however, you can use the desiccated (shredded) kind. To prepare desiccated coconut, simply boil up 300 ml/½ pt/ 1¼ cups of the water needed for the soup, then transfer it to a bowl, stir in 50 g/2 oz desiccated coconut and leave to soak for about 30 minutes. Then use a blender to whiz up the mixture. Add this to the soup at the same time as the coriander (cilantro).

SERVES 4

---

30 ml/2 tbsp cold-pressed extra virgin olive oil

1 large onion, finely chopped

4 garlic cloves, finely chopped

5 cm/2 in piece of fresh root ginger, peeled and grated

2 small red chillis, seeded and chopped

300 ml/½ pt/1¼ cups water

4 lime leaves

2 stalks of lemon grass

15 radishes, trimmed and chopped

75 g/3 oz freshly grated coconut

350 g/12 oz white fish fillets, skinned

30 ml/2 tbsp chopped coriander leaves

30 ml/2 tbsp tamari soy sauce

Coriander or basil leaves, to garnish

1 Heat the oil in a large saucepan.

2 Add the onion, garlic, ginger and chilli and fry (sauté) gently for about 4 minutes until soft, stirring regularly. Do not allow the onion or garlic to colour.

3 Add the water to the pan, along with the lime leaves and lemon grass and simmer for 5 minutes.

4 Add the radishes and coconut, then continue simmering for about 6 minutes.

5 Cut the fish into bite-sized pieces and add to the pan along with the coriander and soy sauce and simmer very gently for 1–2 minutes until the fish is just tender.

6 Serve in individual bowls garnished with coriander or basil leaves.

Scottish Dulse Broth

Sea vegetables such as dulse are excellent additions to a detox programme. This is an adaptation of a traditional seaweed recipe from the Scottish Hebridean Islands. You can buy dulse in dried form from most independent health food stores, although you may have to order it from smaller shops. It really is worth making your own stock for this soup – use cheap white fish or ask your fishmonger for fish trimmings, but make sure they are really good and fresh. For a vegetarian version, use good-quality flavoursome vegetable stock (again, home-made is best; see page 15).

SERVES 4

45 ml/3 tbsp cold-pressed extra virgin olive oil

1 onion, chopped

1 medium carrot, chopped

750 ml/1¼ pts/3 cups water

450 g/1 lb cheap white fish or 700 g/1½ lb fish trimmings

30 ml/2 tbsp cider vinegar

1 bouquet garni sachet

25 g/1 oz dried dulse

200 g/7 oz potatoes, cut into chunks

15 ml/1 tbsp cold-pressed extra virgin olive oil

Freshly ground black pepper

450 ml/¾ pt/2 cups soya or other non-dairy milk

5 ml/1 tsp freshly squeezed lemon juice

Sea salt, to taste

Lemon wedges, to garnish

1 First make the stock. Heat 30 ml/2 tbsp of the olive oil in a frying pan (skillet) and fry (sauté) the onion and carrot until soft but not coloured.

2 Transfer the onion and carrot to a large saucepan along with the water, fish or fish trimmings, cider vinegar and bouquet garni sachet. Bring the saucepan to the boil, then simmer gently for about 30 minutes, skimming the surface to remove any scum.

3 Meanwhile, prepare the other soup ingredients. Put the dulse in a small bowl. Add enough water just to cover it and leave to soak for about 8 minutes.

4 Bring a steamer or a small saucepan of water to the boil and steam or boil the potatoes until just tender.

5 Transfer the potato to a medium bowl, add the remaining olive oil, the dulse and any of the water remaining from soaking the dulse. Mash the ingredients together thoroughly, then season with plenty of freshly ground black pepper.

6 Strain the fish stock and pour into a measuring jug. You should have about 450 ml/¾ pt/2 cups. If you have much more than this, return the stock to the saucepan and boil until it is reduced further, then measure again.

7 Add the milk to the stock in the measuring jug to make about 900 ml/1½ pts/3¾ cups in all. Pour the stock back into the saucepan, then gradually whisk in the potato and dulse mixture, using a fork or a balloon whisk.

8 Stir in the lemon juice, then taste and add more black pepper and a little sea salt, if liked.

9 Reheat, then ladle the piping hot soup into individual dishes and serve garnished with lemon wedges.

STARTERS, LIGHT LUNCHES AND SNACKS

This section contains a selection of delicious light dishes suitable for any time of day. Chèvre with Rocket and Papaya (see page 69) makes a quick tasty lunch dish, served with rice cakes or crisp toasted slices of Detox Loaf (see page 186), while Aubergine and Goats' Cheese Pâté (see page 86) and Nori Maki (see page 76) could grace the most elegant supper party. And if you just want a late-night 'filler', try Tofu Scramble (see page 85).

Chèvre with Rocket and Papaya

Dress the salad immediately before serving; any earlier and the delicate leaves will lose their freshness and crispness.

SERVES 4

Freshly squeezed juice of ½ lemon

Freshly squeezed juice of ½ lime

15 ml/1 tbsp almond or olive oil

5 ml/1 tsp tamari soy sauce

100 g/4 oz chèvre (soft goats' cheese)

1 papaya

50 g/2 oz rocket leaves

50 g/2 oz mixed salad leaves, such as lambs' lettuce, sorrel, little gem, lollo rosso

Freshly ground black pepper

Fresh basil leaves, to garnish

---

1 First make the dressing. Put the lemon and lime juices into a small bowl, add the oil and soy sauce and stir to combine.

2 Slice the chèvre into thin slices, then cut the slices in half.

3 Halve the papaya, scoop out the seeds and any stray fibres, then peel and slice the fruit.

4 Place all the salad leaves in a large bowl, pour over three-quarters of the dressing and toss well.

5 Arrange the leaves on a platter, then arrange the chèvre and papaya on top. Drizzle the rest of the dressing over the cheese and fruit. Season with freshly ground black pepper and garnish with basil leaves, then serve immediately.

Mixed Melon Starter

A good summer recipe when melons are plentiful, sweet and cheap. The delicate combination of white and pale green fruit creates a pretty colour contrast and melon is an excellent cleansing food, as is its natural partner, ginger. For a change, instead of the marinated tofu, try using sliced Feta cheese, sprinkled with fresh grated root ginger (omit the lemon juice and soy sauce), before refrigerating. If you have an especially sensitive digestion, you should avoid combining melon with other foods while following a detox programme, so omit the cucumber, tofu and soy, and toss the melon balls in ginger before serving.

SERVES 4

200 g/7 oz block of smoked or natural tofu

3 cm/1¼ in piece of fresh root ginger, peeled and grated

Freshly squeezed juice of 1 lemon

30 ml/2 tbsp tamari soy sauce

3 cm/1¼ in piece of cucumber

½ medium honeydew melon, chilled

½ cantaloupe melon, chilled

1.5 ml/¼ tsp paprika

1 Dry the block of tofu thoroughly with kitchen paper (paper towels), blotting to remove excess liquid. Cut into 5 mm/¼ in slices and arrange in a shallow dish.

2 Place the grated ginger, lemon juice and soy sauce in a small bowl and stir to combine. Pour over the tofu, cover and refrigerate for at least an hour (overnight is ideal).

3   Remove the seeds from the melon halves, then make small balls using a melon baller. Alternatively, remove the melon flesh from the skin and cut into neat 2 cm/ ¾ in cubes. Arrange the melon balls in four individual dishes.

4   Remove the tofu from the fridge and drain if necessary (do not remove the grated ginger from the surface). Cut into matchsticks.

5   Cut the cucumber into matchsticks (do not remove the skin – it will add colour contrast and crunchy texture to the dish).

6   Arrange the tofu and the cucumber in a radiating pattern in the four glasses. Add a pinch of paprika to the centre of each glass and serve.

Papaya and Pineapple

This starter looks very attractive if you alternate the orange papaya slices and the pale yellow pineapple on the plate. You can't get more detox than this dish – both pineapple and papaya are packed with useful enzymes.

SERVES 4

1 medium pineapple

2 papayas

2 cm/¾ in piece of root ginger

Freshly squeezed juice of ½ lemon

Freshly ground black pepper

A few small lollo rosso lettuce leaves, to garnish

1 Peel the pineapple and slice it neatly, then halve each slice. Remove the core if it is woody.

2 Halve the papayas, scoop out the seeds and any stray fibres, then carefully peel and slice the fruit.

3 Arrange alternating slices of pineapple and papaya on individual plates.

4 Peel the ginger and place in a garlic press. Squeeze the juice from the ginger root over the fruit, taking care not to drop any solid matter.

5 Pour the lemon juice over the fruit, then season with freshly ground black pepper.

6 Garnish each plate with a leaf or two of lollo rosso, then serve.

Asparagus with Tahini Dressing

Asparagus is considered by detox nutritionists to be one of the best kidney cleansers, ideally eaten raw or lightly cooked. Here it is very lightly steamed, and served with a creamy dressing made from tahini (sesame seed paste). Sesame seeds are not only rich in vitamins and minerals, but are also thought to be useful in helping to regulate cholesterol in the body.

SERVES 4 AS A STARTER

20–24 asparagus spears, trimmed

60 ml/4 tbsp light tahini

15 ml/1 tbsp freshly squeezed lemon juice

60 ml/4 tbsp fresh apple juice

1 garlic clove, crushed

5 ml/1 tsp tamari soy sauce

5 ml/1 tsp cold-pressed extra virgin olive oil

5 ml/1 tsp chopped marjoram

Freshly ground black pepper

A few drops of freshly squeezed lemon juice, to taste

Sprigs of marjoram, to garnish

1 Bring a steamer to boiling point and then place the asparagus in the steamer. Cook for 3–4 minutes, no more.

2 Whisk together the tahini, lemon and apple juices, garlic, soy sauce, olive oil and chopped marjoram for the dressing.

3 Divide the asparagus spears between four warmed individual plates, season with black pepper and a little extra lemon juice, garnish with sprigs of marjoram and serve immediately with a dish of the tahini dressing.

Afghani-style Aubergine with Yoghurt Dressing

SERVES 4

30 ml/2 tbsp cold-pressed extra virgin olive oil

1 aubergine (eggplant), about 550 g/1¼ lb, sliced

25 g/1 oz/¼ cup millet

25 g/1 oz/¼ cup almonds

1 small onion, chopped

1 small garlic clove, crushed

2.5 ml/½ tsp freshly squeezed lemon juice

7.5 ml/1½ tsp tamari soy sauce

1 cm/½ in piece of root ginger

1.5 ml/¼ tsp ground cinnamon

2.5 ml/½ tsp ground cumin

2.5 ml/½ tsp ground coriander (cilantro)

1.5 ml/¼ tsp hot paprika

2 green cardamoms, peeled

150 ml/¼ pt/⅔ cup Yoghurt Dressing (see page 75)

Sprigs of marjoram, to garnish

1   Heat 15 ml/1 tbsp of the oil in a large frying pan (skillet) and cook the aubergine slices for about 1 minute on each side until softened slightly.

2   Cook the millet in about 300 ml/½ pt/1¼ cups boiling water for 5–6 minutes until softened. Drain and place in a medium mixing bowl.

3 Put the almonds, onion, garlic, lemon juice, soy sauce, 15 ml/1 tbsp olive oil and all the spices in a blender.

4 Blend to a medium-fine consistency, then stir into the millet until thoroughly combined.

5 Place 10–15 ml/2–3 tsp stuffing on each slice of aubergine, then fold over. Put the stuffed aubergine rolls into an oiled ovenproof dish, arranging them snugly against each other so they do not unroll. Drizzle a little more oil over the top, then bake in a preheated oven at 190°C/375°F/gas mark 5 for about 30 minutes.

6 Place three or four aubergine slices on each individual plate, add a dollop of Yoghurt Dressing and garnish with sprigs of marjoram before serving.

Yoghurt Dressing

This is a useful dressing for salads and also for fish dishes, especially if you replace the marjoram with dill (dill weed) or finely chopped fennel. To make a stronger flavoured dressing, add a little finely crushed garlic.

MAKES ABOUT 150 ML/¼ PT/⅔ CUP

150 ml/¼ pt/⅔ cup live goats', sheep's or soya yoghurt

10 ml/2 tsp chopped marjoram

A few drops of freshly squeezed lemon juice (optional)

A little paprika

Marjoram leaves, to garnish

1 Place the yoghurt in a medium bowl. Stir in the marjoram.

2 If the yoghurt is very mild, use a few drops of lemon to sharpen the flavour.

3 Sprinkle with paprika and garnish with marjoram leaves.

Nori Maki

These extremely elegant little Japanese appetisers are made from rice and vegetables rolled up in a sheet of Japanese laver seaweed. Simple to make, this version is also excellent for your detox programme. You can buy sheets of Japanese laver seaweed (nori) from health food stores, ready-toasted or untoasted. Before using untoasted sheets, pass them rapidly back and forth over a flame (about 20 cm/8 in away) until the sheet turns from black to green.

SERVES 4

---

100 g/4 oz/½ cup round wholegrain rice

250 ml/8 fl oz/1 cup water

20 ml/4 tsp cider vinegar

Sea salt

4 dark green lettuce leaves, thick stalks removed

2.5 ml/½ tsp tamari soy sauce

A few drops of freshly squeezed lemon juice

2 sheets of toasted Japanese laver seaweed

1 small red (bell) pepper, cut into matchsticks

1 medium carrot, cut into matchsticks

1   Put the rice and the water in a saucepan with a tight-fitting lid. Bring to the boil, cover, then simmer for about 15–18 minutes. Remove the saucepan from the heat, and set aside for 5 minutes, leaving the lid on. The rice should then be soft and all the water absorbed.

2   Transfer the rice to a mixing bowl, add the vinegar and a little sea salt and mix well.

3 Bring a steamer or a small saucepan of water to the boil. Place the lettuce leaves in the steamer or saucepan of boiling water and cook for 20–30 seconds, until the leaves are wilted.

4 Transfer the lettuce leaves to a small bowl, add the soy sauce and lemon juice and finely chop the leaves.

5 Lay a sheet of toasted Japanese laver on greaseproof (waxed) paper. Spread half the rice over the laver, leaving a 5 cm/2 in margin along the edge furthest away from you.

6 Arrange half the carrot sticks end to end along the centre of the sheet, parallel to the uncovered top margin of laver, then half the pepper sticks in the same way alongside. Next, arrange half the chopped lettuce running parallel to the carrot and pepper.

7 Carefully roll up the sheet of laver like a Swiss (jelly) roll, working from the edge nearest to you to the top uncovered edge.

8 Dampen the uncovered edge with a little water and seal firmly.

9 Repeat steps 5–8 to make a second roll.

10 With a sharp, wet knife, cut the two rolls into 2 cm/ ¾ in slices and serve cold or steam for a few minutes and serve warm.

Crudités with Creamy Tofu Dip

Marjoram adds a pleasantly sweet Mediterranean flavour to this starter, but you can use any herbs you like – experiment with your favourite varieties. Restrict yourself to two or three different kinds at one time, however, or the flavours will become indistinct.

SERVES 4

150 g/5 oz/generous ½ cup tofu, drained and cubed

40 ml/2½ tbsp cold-pressed extra virgin olive oil

40 ml/2½ tbsp fresh apple juice, plus a little more if necessary

2.5 ml/½ tsp cider vinegar

1 small garlic clove, crushed

5 ml/1 tsp chopped rosemary

5 ml/1 tsp chopped marjoram

A pinch of English mustard powder

Freshly ground black pepper

2 large carrots, cut into sticks

½ small cucumber, cut into sticks

2 celery sticks, cut into short lengths

Sprigs of marjoram, to garnish

1 Place the tofu in a blender with the olive oil, apple juice, cider vinegar, garlic, chopped herbs and mustard powder and blend for about 30 seconds until smooth and creamy.

2 Test the consistency. If it is too stiff, add a little more apple juice. Season with freshly ground black pepper and blend again for a few seconds.

3 Transfer to a covered dish and refrigerate for about 30 minutes or until needed.

5 Arrange the carrot, cucumber and celery sticks around a bowl of the dip on a large serving platter, and garnish the dip with the marjoram sprigs. Alternatively, serve individual plates of crudités and dip.

Hazelnut and Lemon Butter

This is an ideal lunchtime filling for Detox Loaf (see page 186) or rice cakes and makes an excellent starter or teatime snack. You can vary the flavours by adding herbs, or a little garlic or chilli, if you like. It will keep in a screw-topped jar in the fridge for a few days.

SERVES 2
---

100 g/4 oz/1 cup hazelnuts (filberts)

20 ml/4 tsp cold-pressed extra virgin olive oil

10 ml/2 tsp freshly squeezed lemon juice

A little herb salt or sea salt, to taste

1 Place all the ingredients except the salt in a food processor and process for about 20 seconds to create a fairly fine consistency.

2 Taste and add a little herb salt or sea salt, if necessary, then process again for a few seconds.

3 Serve spread on rice cakes or thin slices of Detox Loaf, toasted if you prefer.

Hummus with Crudités

You don't have to use kombu seaweed to cook the chick peas (garbanzos) in this recipe but it does reduce the cooking time and help to make the chick peas more digestible. Like all seaweeds, kombu is full of nutrients, and is considered to be a great detoxer.

SERVES 4

---

175 g/6 oz dried chick peas

1 strip of kombu seaweed (optional)

15 ml/1 tbsp cold-pressed extra virgin olive oil

40 ml/2½ tbsp tahini (sesame seed paste)

30–40 ml/1–2 tbsp water, if needed

Freshly ground black pepper

Freshly squeezed juice of 1½–2 lemons

1–2 large garlic cloves, crushed

12 green beans

2 good-sized carrots, cut into thin sticks

2 celery sticks, cut into thin short lengths

1 red (bell) pepper, cut into thin strips

8 spring onions (scallions), trimmed

12–15 stoned (pitted) black olives, for garnish

---

1 Rinse the chick peas, then place them in a bowl and cover with water. Leave them in a cool place to soak for about 3 hours, or overnight.

2 Drain the chick peas, and place them in a saucepan with plenty of water. Add the kombu and bring to the boil. (If the kombu bobs to the surface, push it down into the water again.) Boil the chick peas for 2 minutes, then skim off any scum. Turn down the heat and simmer until the chick peas are tender (about 30 minutes).

3 Remove from the heat. Remove the kombu and set it aside for garnishing, if you like. Drain and rinse the chick peas.

4 Put the chick peas, olive oil, tahini, 15 ml/1 tbsp water and a generous grinding of black pepper in a food processor, adding lemon juice and garlic to taste.

5 Process the ingredients to a smooth consistency. If the mixture becomes too thick, add a little more water.

6 Taste and adjust the seasoning. You may want to add more lemon juice or garlic, then process for a minute or two longer.

7 Next, prepare the crudités. Plunge the beans in a pan of boiling water for about 30 seconds, then drain and plunge in cold water. Arrange all the crudités on a platter with a bowl of hummus in the centre.

8 Garnish with black olives and finely shredded kombu, if liked.

Olive, Sweet Pepper and Hazelnut Pâté

This tasty nut pâté can be eaten as a starter with crudités or rice cakes, or used as a lunchtime sandwich filling between thin slices of Detox Loaf (see page 186). Store it in a screw-topped jar in the fridge if you are using it as a sandwich filling, but don't keep it for more than a couple of days – detox food should always be eaten as fresh as possible.

SERVES 4 AS A STARTER

---

1 medium red (bell) pepper, cut into 8 pieces

1 medium green pepper, cut into 8 pieces

45 ml/3 tbsp cold-pressed extra virgin olive oil

75 g/3 oz/¾ cup hazelnuts (filberts)

50 g/2 oz stoned (pitted) black olives

1 garlic clove, crushed

¼ onion, chopped

5 ml/1 tsp chopped oregano,

A few drops of freshly squeezed lemon juice

A few drops of tamari soy sauce

Freshly ground black pepper

Sea salt, to taste

---

1 Place the peppers on a roasting tray and drizzle 15 ml/ 1 tbsp olive oil over them.

2 Roast the peppers in a preheated oven at 190°C/375°F/gas mark 5 for about 30 minutes, basting occasionally, until tender and well browned.

3 Remove the peppers from the roasting tray and set aside. Add the hazelnuts to the tray, rolling them in any remaining olive oil.

4 Roast the nuts in the oven for about 6 minutes until just golden brown, shaking the tray once during this time.

5 Place the peppers, nuts, olives, garlic, onion, oregano and the remaining olive oil in a blender and whiz for about 10 seconds. If the mixture is too stiff, add a little water.

6 Scrape around the goblet, add the lemon juice, soy sauce and a generous grinding of black pepper and blend the mixture for a further 15 seconds or so, until the mixture is reduced to a coarse pâté consistency. (I like it with recognisable pieces of nut, olive and pepper dotted through the mixture.)

7 Test for seasoning and stir in a little sea salt, if necessary.

Savoury Toasts with Alfalfa Topping

This is an excellent speedy starter, and also makes a useful light lunch dish, perhaps with a bowl of soup or a salad. The savoury spread, incidentally, is also good as a tasty topping for vegetables. Try to buy organic tahini if you can. You will find both light and the stronger flavoured dark tahini in your local health food store, as you will alfalfa sprouts, although these are easy to grow yourself (see page 20).

SERVES 4

8 slices of Detox Loaf (see page 186)

60 ml/4 tbsp light tahini

10 ml/2 tsp freshly squeezed lemon juice

20 ml/4 tsp tamari soy sauce

15 ml/1 tbsp finely chopped red onion

15 ml/1 tbsp chopped basil

60 ml/4 tbsp alfalfa sprouts

1 Toast the slices of bread. Place in a toast rack to keep crisp until required.

2 Put the tahini, lemon juice, soy sauce, onion and basil in a bowl and stir well to combine them.

3 Cut each slice of toast into two triangles, then spread thickly with the savoury spread. Top each triangle with a couple of generous pinches of alfalfa sprouts and serve immediately.

Tofu Scramble

I like to pile this savoury scramble on rice cakes, as a starter or a quick lunch, but it's also excellent heated in a frying pan (skillet) with a little extra olive oil.

SERVES 4 AS A STARTER

20 ml/4 tsp tamari soy sauce

20 ml/4 tsp cold-pressed extra virgin olive oil

2.5 ml/½ tsp grated nutmeg

7.5 ml/1½ tsp freshly squeezed lemon juice

350 g/12 oz/1½ cups firm tofu

A few sprigs of flatleaf parsley or chives, for garnish

1 Put the soy sauce, oil, nutmeg and lemon juice into a bowl.

2 Add the tofu and mash it into the other ingredients, stirring well to combine all the flavours.

3 Serve with rice cakes or thin toasted slices of Detox Loaf (see page 186), garnished with parsley or chives.

Aubergine and Goats' Cheese Pâté

Many recipes recommend sprinkling salt over slices of aubergine (eggplant) before cooking them, to draw out bitter juices and excess water. This is not really necessary and should be avoided if you are making detox dishes and trying to reduce salt content to a minimum.

SERVES 4 AS A STARTER

45 ml/3 tbsp cold-pressed extra virgin olive oil

45 ml/3 tbsp rice flour

1 aubergine, sliced

1 fat garlic clove, crushed

50 g/2 oz soft mild goats' cheese

A little freshly squeezed lemon juice

Freshly ground black pepper

Herb salt or sea salt, to taste

1 Put the rice flour in a shallow dish. Press the aubergine slices into the flour to coat both sides thoroughly.

2 Heat the olive oil in a large frying pan (skillet) and fry (sauté) the aubergine slices, turning once to ensure they are soft and cooked through. (You may find it easiest to cook them in batches.)

3 When all the aubergine slices are cooked, place them in a food processor along with the garlic and goats' cheese. Process to a medium consistency – there should still be some texture to the pâté.

4 Taste and season carefully with lemon juice, black pepper and a little herb salt or sea salt, if necessary.

5 Serve with toasted slices of Detox Loaf (see page 186), rice cakes or crudités.

Savoury Sunflower Seeds

Nuts and seeds make a delicious snack or addition to a lunch box. In this recipe, sunflower seeds are tossed in tamari soy sauce before being gently cooked in the oven. Substitute pine nuts for sunflower seeds if you like, although these are rather richer and you will probably need fewer of them.

SERVES 4 AS A SNACK

100 g/4 oz/1 cup sunflower seeds

10 ml/2 tsp tamari soy sauce

5 ml/1 tsp freshly squeezed lemon juice

1 Place the sunflower seeds, soy sauce and lemon juice in a medium bowl and mix all the ingredients thoroughly to coat the seeds.

2 Spread the seeds out on a baking (cookie) sheet and bake in a preheated oven at 160°C/350°F/gas mark 3 for about 10 minutes, turning once or twice during cooking.

3 Remove from the oven, spoon on to a plate and leave to cool before serving.

SALADS AND SALAD DRESSINGS

Tasty salads are at the heart of any good detox diet, offering a wealth of nutrients, tastes, colours and textures in a huge variety of fresh, raw ingredients. And they need never be boring – a delicious dressing can transform even the most ordinary ingredients. All the dressings in this book are designed to be useful additions to your detox programme, so you don't need stint yourself. Experiment with different dressing and salad combinations – the possibilities are almost endless!

Mixed Green Salad

You can make endless delicious variations on the green salad theme – just include your favourite herbs and salad leaves plus whatever looks good and fresh in the shops and the garden, mixing them in whatever proportions you like. Use any of the salad dressings included in this book, or no dressing at all. A simple sprinkling of fresh lemon juice and olive oil is quick, easy and very tasty.

SERVES 4
---

100 g/4 oz mixed herb and salad greens using any of the following:

rocket
lettuce varieties – mix several varieties of differently coloured and shaped leaves;
finely shredded cabbage;
Chinese leaves (stem lettuce);
spring onions (scallions);
finely shredded leek;
fennel;
nasturtium leaves;
watercress;
cress, rape, mustard and other growing salads;
alfalfa, moong and other sprouts;
celery leaves;
snipped chives;
basil, parsley, coriander (cilantro), marjoram or oregano;
very finely chopped rosemary and thyme;
lovage;
chervil;
raw mangetout (snow peas), sugarsnaps or finely chopped green beans

Tear the leaves roughly and toss all your chosen ingredients together, with or without a dressing, then serve.

Fruity Coleslaw

The red skins of the apples create a pretty colour contrast in this sweet, crunchy salad.

SERVES 4

⅓ head white cabbage, stalk removed

2 medium carrots, grated

1½ small crisp red eating (dessert) apples

½ onion, finely chopped

15 ml/1 tbsp freshly squeezed lemon juice

30 ml/2 tbsp fresh apple juice

75 ml/5 tbsp Detox Mayonnaise (see page 91)

Freshly ground black pepper

6–8 basil leaves

1 Finely shred the cabbage and place in a large bowl together with the grated carrot and chopped onion.

2 Core one apple, then very finely chop it and add it to the cabbage, carrot and onion.

3 Sprinkle over 10 ml/2 tsp lemon juice, then toss the ingredients to mix and coat them in the juice.

4 Place the apple juice and Detox Mayonnaise in a small bowl and mix thoroughly. Season with black pepper.

5 Add to the cabbage mixture and toss thoroughly.

6 Roughly tear up all but two of the basil leaves and stir into the coleslaw.

7 Core and thinly slice the remaining half apple, dip the slices in the remaining lemon juice to prevent them discolouring, then use to garnish the salad with the remaining basil leaves.

Detox Mayonnaise

This creamy all-purpose salad dressing contains nutmeg which helps to stimulate appetite and digestion when added to food – but don't overdo this spice when following a detox diet. The mayonnaise is best made in small quantities as you need it, although it will keep for a couple of days in a screw-topped jar in the fridge.

MAKES 150 ML/¼ PT/⅔ CUP

150 g/5 oz/generous ½ cup tofu, cut into cubes

60 ml/4 tbsp cold-pressed extra virgin olive oil

7.5 ml/1½ tsp cider vinegar

20 ml/4 tsp fresh apple juice

5 ml/1 tsp English mustard powder

1 garlic clove, crushed

2.5 ml/½ tsp chopped French tarragon

Freshly ground black pepper

Sea salt

Freshly grated nutmeg

1 Place the tofu in a blender.

2 Add the olive oil, vinegar, apple juice, mustard, garlic and tarragon to the blender and blend for about 10 seconds. Remove the blender lid, scrape the contents to the bottom of the goblet, then blend again for about 20 seconds, until the mixture is smooth and creamy.

3 If the mayonnaise seems too thick, add a little more apple juice and blend again for a few seconds.

4 Season with freshly ground black pepper, a little sea salt and some freshly grated nutmeg. Blend again for a few seconds.

5 Transfer to a screw-topped jar and refrigerate until required.

California Salad with Citrus Dressing

Creamy avocados complement the tang of citrus and the richness of walnuts in this brilliantly coloured and refreshing salad. The onions, grapes, celery and olive oil are all great detoxers while avocados gently encourage the digestive system to work efficiently. Avocados are rich in natural oils but easy to digest – they are given to small babies as a weaning food in some parts of the world.

SERVES 4
---

1 carrot, cut into matchsticks

2 celery sticks, cut into matchsticks

2 medium oranges

20 seedless grapes

3 spring onions (scallions), finely chopped

1 avocado, peeled and stoned (pitted)

75 g/3 oz/¾ cup walnut halves

1 quantity of Citrus Dressing (see page 93)

1 Put the carrot and celery in a large bowl.

2 Peel the oranges and cut them up, removing any pips, then add to the bowl with the grapes and the spring onions. Chop the avocado flesh and add to the bowl.

3 Taste one of the walnut halves. If the skin is bitter, drop the nuts into a pan of boiling water for about 10 seconds to loosen the skins. Then drain them and rub them vigorously in a tea towel (dish cloth) to remove most of the skins, or peel off the skins with your fingers.

4 Add the nuts to the salad, then pour over the Citrus Dressing and toss thoroughly.

Citrus Dressing

Freshly squeezed juice of 1 medium orange

30 ml/2 tbsp walnut oil

15 ml/1 tbsp cold-pressed extra virgin olive oil

5 ml/1 tsp freshly squeezed lemon juice

1 whole garlic clove

A splash of tamari soy sauce

Freshly ground black pepper

1 Put the orange juice into a small bowl.

2 Add the two oils and lemon juice to the bowl. Crush the garlic clove in a garlic press and add only the juice to the dressing, then add the soy sauce and black pepper and stir thoroughly. Leave for about 30 minutes in a cool place for the flavours to develop.

Rice and Cashew Nut Salad with Lime Dressing

You can adjust the spiciness of this saffron-yellow salad by varying the amount of chilli. This dish is, incidentally, just as good served hot as cold and makes an excellent main course served with a green leaf salad or a green vegetable.

SERVES 4–6 AS A SIDE DISH

---

100 g/4 oz/1 cup round wholegrain rice

2.5 cm/1 in piece of cinnamon stick or 2 small pieces of cassia bark

2 green cardamoms

250 ml/8 fl oz/1 cup water

50 g/2 oz green beans

30 ml/2 tbsp cold-pressed extra virgin olive oil

1 small onion, finely chopped

1 garlic clove, crushed

2.5 cm/1 in piece of ginger root, grated

½ small chilli, seeded and chopped

½ red (bell) pepper, sliced

50 g/2 oz/½ cup cashew nuts

1 medium carrot, cut into matchsticks

1 spring onion (scallion), cut into matchsticks

Freshly squeezed juice of ½ lime

A few drops of freshly squeezed lemon juice

A pinch of saffron

15 ml/1 tbsp chopped flatleaf parsley, plus a few leaves to garnish

1 Put the rice, cinnamon or cassia bark, cardamoms and water in a saucepan and cover with a tight-fitting lid. Bring to the boil, then simmer for 15–18 minutes. Remove the saucepan from the heat and set aside, leaving the lid on.

2 Meanwhile, steam or boil the green beans until cooked but still very firm. Plunge instantly into cold water to help retain their colour and texture, then drain and set aside.

3 Heat the olive oil in a large frying pan (skillet) and fry (sauté) the onion and garlic for about 4 minutes.

4 Stir the ginger and chilli into the pan, then continue cooking for a further 4 minutes.

5 Stir the pepper into the onion mixture along with the cashew nuts and cook for a further 3 minutes. Remove the pan from the heat.

6 Put the carrots and spring onion in a large bowl with the green beans.

7 Remove the cardamoms and cinnamon or cassia bark from the rice, then stir the rice into the onion mixture.

8 Sprinkle the lime and lemon juices over the carrots, spring onion and green beans, then stir into the rice mixture, ensuring that all the ingredients are thoroughly combined.

9 Immediately before serving, stir in the saffron and chopped parsley and garnish with parsley leaves.

Feta, Olive and Summer Herb Salad

Add your own favourite salad herbs to this dish, but try to include sorrel, for its sharp lemony flavour, and plenty of spicy-tasting rocket. Rocket, incidentally, is astonishingly easy to grow in the garden and transforms any summer salad. Replace the Feta with home-made Tofu Cheese (see page 98) if you are avoiding dairy products altogether. Double the quantities to serve this dish as a main course salad for four.

SERVES 4 AS A SIDE DISH

450 g/1 lb new potatoes, scrubbed

1 yellow (bell) pepper, cut into quarters

4 tender sorrel leaves

75 g/3 oz mangetout (snow peas) or sugar snap peas

12 basil leaves

15 ml/1 tbsp chopped sweet marjoram

A handful of rocket leaves

A handful of mixed salad leaves, such as lambs' lettuce, chervil, salad burnet, purslane and other lettuce varieties

20 black olives, stoned (pitted)

100 g/4 oz/1 cup Feta cheese, cut into small cubes

20 ml/4 tbsp Oil and Vinegar Dressing (see page 97)

1 Steam or boil the potatoes in their skins until tender. Set aside until cool enough to handle.

2 Meanwhile, place the pepper quarters on a grill (broiler) pan under a preheated grill and cook until the skin is well coloured and the flesh is soft. Set aside.

3 Roughly tear the sorrel leaves and place in a large bowl. Add the mangetout or sugar snap peas, basil leaves, marjoram, other salad leaves and olives.

4 Add the Feta cubes to the salad bowl.

5 Cut the warm potatoes into 2 cm/¾ in pieces and the pepper into 1 cm/½ in squares. Add these to the salad bowl.

6 Pour 25 ml/1½ tbsp Oil and Vinegar Dressing over the salad and toss well before serving.

Oil and Vinegar Dressing

This is a basic vinaigrette-style dressing. Add a little crushed garlic, finely chopped shallot, dry mustard powder, finely chopped herbs or a few drops of tamari soy sauce to vary it, or try substituting one-third of the cider vinegar with balsamic vinegar.

MAKES 55 ML/3½ TBSP

45 ml/3 tbsp cold-pressed extra virgin olive oil

15 ml/1 tbsp cider vinegar

Freshly ground black pepper

1 Put the oil and cider vinegar in a small jug along with a generous grinding of freshly ground black pepper.

2 Stir thoroughly to combine.

Tofu Cheese

This makes an excellent non-dairy substitute for the Feta in the Feta, Olive and Summer Herb Salad (see page 96). Follow the same recipe instructions, but add 175 g/6 oz/1½ cups Tofu Cheese, cut into bite-sized pieces, instead of the Feta. Make the Tofu Cheese at least 2 hours in advance, or preferably the day before, to allow the flavours to penetrate the tofu.

SERVES 2–4

---

175 g/6 oz block of tofu

15 ml/1 tbsp tamari soy sauce

½ small onion, very finely chopped

10 ml/2 tsp freshly squeezed lemon juice

---

1 Wrap the tofu block in a clean tea towel (dish cloth) and place a weight on it to squeeze out all the excess water. Leave for at least 15 minutes.

2 Unwrap the block and slice the tofu, blotting each slice with kitchen paper (paper towels) to remove any remaining water. Arrange the slices in a shallow dish.

3 Put the soy sauce in a small bowl with the chopped onion and the lemon juice. Stir to combine all the ingredients.

4 Pour the soy sauce mixture over the tofu, making sure all the slices are coated on both sides.

5 Set aside in a cool place for at least 2 hours to allow the flavours to combine before using it.

Beetroot and Pear Salad

Beetroot (red beet) is considered to be one of the best cleansing foods, especially if eaten raw. Its sweet earthiness combines well with the creaminess of the mayonnaise, which it turns a fabulous magenta colour. Try to buy rosy-skinned pears for this salad to create a brilliant red plate of colour.

SERVES 4

1 medium beetroot, about 150 g/5 oz, scrubbed

2 spring onions (scallions), finely chopped

100 ml/3½ fl oz/scant ½ cup Detox Mayonnaise (see page 91) or Creamy Salad Dressing (see page 112)

1 sweetheart, little gem or other small lettuce

2 red-skinned pears, cored and sliced

Freshly squeezed juice of ½ lemon

Freshly ground black pepper

Sea salt

1 Grate the beetroot into a medium bowl.

2 Add the chopped spring onions to the bowl with the Detox Mayonnaise or Creamy Salad Dressing. Stir thoroughly to combine.

3 Arrange the beetroot mixture in the middle of a large platter and arrange the lettuce leaves around it.

4 Dip the pear slices in the lemon juice and arrange on the platter.

5 Sprinkle a little of the remaining lemon juice over the salad, then season with freshly ground black pepper and a little sea salt.

Icelandic Beetroot and Haddock Salad with Mustard Dressing

This is a detox version of a traditional Icelandic dish. The haddock is served cold, which might seem odd, but is surprisingly delicious providing you are very careful not to overcook the fish.
You can buy dried dulse from most independent health food stores, though you may have to order it.

SERVES 4

2 medium beetroot (red beets), preferably raw

75 ml/5 tbsp cider vinegar

½ cucumber

Sea salt

100 g/4 oz/¾ cup fine millet flakes

30 ml/2 tbsp freshly squeezed lemon juice

30 ml/2 tbsp water

45 ml/3 tbsp cold-pressed extra virgin olive oil

450 g/1 lb fresh haddock fillets

200 ml/7 fl oz/scant 1 cup Mustard Dressing (see page 102)

4 spring onions (scallions)

1 bunch of watercress or 2 boxes of growing cress

45 ml/3 tbsp chopped parsley

15 g/½ oz dried dulse

1 Scrub the beetroot, then boil or steam until just tender. Set aside until cool, then peel and slice.

2 Arrange in a shallow dish and pour over 45 ml/3 tbsp cider vinegar. Leave in a cool place for at least 2 hours.

3 Slice the cucumber and arrange on a plate. Sprinkle sea salt over it and leave for about 30 minutes.

4 Rinse the cucumber and squeeze it dry, then arrange it in a shallow dish and pour the remaining 30 ml/2 tbsp cider vinegar over it. Leave it in a cool place for at least 2 hours.

5 Mix together the millet flakes, 5 ml/1 tsp lemon juice, the water and 30 ml/2 tbsp olive oil, so that the ingredients stick together to form a dough.

6 Lightly oil a set of small bun tins (patty pans), then press the millet mixture firmly into the tins to form eight to ten thin, cup-shaped croustades.

7 Put the croustades in a preheated oven at 160°C/325°F/gas mark 3 for about 25 minutes until crisp. When they are removed from the oven, let them cool slightly before removing them from the tins.

8 To prepare the haddock, sprinkle 10 ml/2 tsp lemon juice over the fish, and season lightly with a little sea salt. Steam the fish very gently in a steamer or on a covered plate over a saucepan of boiling water for about 4 minutes, until the flesh turns opaque and flakes easily. Be very careful not to overcook it. Set aside to cool, then cut into neat pieces.

9 Drain the beetroot, then chop finely and place into a medium bowl. Drain and chop the cucumber and add to the bowl together with the Mustard Dressing and mix thoroughly.

10 Finely chop the spring onions and place in a large bowl with the watercress or growing cress and the parsley. Add 15 ml/1 tbsp olive oil and 15 ml/1 tbsp lemon juice and toss well. Arrange on a large serving platter with the haddock pieces garnished with dulse, snipped into slivers.

11 Fill the croustades with the beetroot mixture and arrange these on the platter too with any leftover beetroot mixture piled in the middle.

Mustard Dressing

This creamy dressing is good with bean salads and all kinds of fish, or try it drizzled over corn on the cob. You can make it up to a day in advance.

MAKES ABOUT 450 ML/¾ PT/2 CUPS

45 ml/3 tbsp cold-pressed extra virgin olive oil

30 ml/2 tbsp wholemeal rice flour

10 ml/2 tsp English mustard powder

300 ml/½ pt/1¼ cups soya milk

1 whole garlic clove

5 ml/1 tsp tamari soy sauce

25 ml/5 tsp fresh apple juice

45 ml/3 tbsp cider vinegar

2.5ml/½ tsp freshly squeezed lemon juice

10 ml/2 tsp wholegrain mustard

Freshly ground black pepper

Sea salt, to taste

1 Heat the olive oil in a frying pan (skillet), then carefully stir in the rice flour and mustard powder. Gradually add the soya milk, stirring continuously and cook, stirring, until the mixture thickens.

2 Crush the garlic clove in a garlic press and add a few drops of the garlic juice to the pan. Do not allow any solid matter to fall into the pan.

3 Add the soy sauce and very carefully stir in the apple juice and the cider vinegar, stirring continuously to prevent the mixture curdling.

4 Stir in the lemon juice and wholegrain mustard, then test for seasoning and add freshly ground black pepper, and a little sea salt, if necessary.

6 Set aside to cool. As it cools, stir vigorously every now and again to prevent it congealing. If it seems to be getting too sticky, use a balloon whisk or fork to whisk in a little more soya milk. Once cool, it should have a smooth, thick, pouring consistency.

Vegetable Salad with Leeks, Celeriac and Broad Beans

This is a marvellously satisfying salad dish, combining a mixture of raw and cooked vegetables. Make sure the cooked vegetables still have plenty of bite left in them for maximum colour and crunch.

SERVES 4

275 g/10 oz potatoes, cut into chunks

2 large carrots, cut into chunks

150 g/5 oz broccoli, broken into small florets

1 medium leek, sliced

150 g/5 oz celeriac (celery root)

150 g/5 oz baby broad (fava) beans

250 ml/8 fl oz/1 cup Tofu, Lemon and Parsley Dressing (see page 105)

1 Boil or, ideally, steam the potato and carrot chunks until they are only just cooked. They can be cooked together in the same pan but the potatoes will need longer cooking time and should be firm but tender; the carrots should be barely cooked. As soon as they are done, plunge them into cold water, drain and set aside to cool.

2 Steam or boil the broccoli florets for about 3 minutes and as soon as they are cooked, plunge them under cold water, drain and set aside to cool.

3 Steam or gently boil the broad beans until they are tender. Do not overcook them or their skins will become leathery. Drain and set aside.

4 Heat the oil in a frying pan (skillet) and fry (sauté) the leek until slightly softened. Remove from the pan with a slotted spoon and transfer to a large bowl.

5 Grate the celeriac into the bowl with the leek. Cut the potatoes into neat 2 cm/¾ in pieces and add to the bowl, together with the carrot, cut into neat 1 cm/½ in pieces, and the broccoli florets.

6 Pour the Tofu, Parsley and Lemon Dressing over the salad and toss well.

Tofu, Parsley and Lemon Dressing

The parsley, lemon juice and olive oil in this salad are all considered excellent detoxers.

MAKES ABOUT 300 ML/½ PT/1¼ CUPS

45 ml/3 tbsp cold-pressed extra virgin olive oil

1 garlic clove, crushed

120 g/4½ oz tofu

45 ml/3 tbsp non-dairy milk

45 ml/3 tbsp roughly chopped parsley

7.5 ml/1½ tsp freshly squeezed lemon juice

Freshly ground black pepper

Sea salt or herb salt

1 Heat the oil in a frying pan (skillet). Add the garlic and fry (sauté) it gently until it is softened but not coloured.

2 Cut up the tofu and put it in a blender with the milk. Blend for about 10 seconds to a thick purée.

3 Stir the tofu purée into the garlic and olive oil in the frying pan, then stir in the parsley and lemon juice.

4 Season with freshly ground black pepper and a little sea salt or herb salt.

Fragrant Rice Salad

This delicately spiced salad is created from an unusual combination of fruit and vegetables. If you don't have fresh grapes, raisins taste just as good. You will find lime leaves in oriental stores and large supermarkets.

SERVES 4

225 g/8 oz/1 cup round wholegrain rice

450 ml/¾ pt/2 cups water

2 cardamoms

1 piece of cassia bark or 2 cm/¾ in piece of cinnamon stick

2 lime leaves (optional)

50 g/2 oz green beans

½ red onion, sliced

½ yellow or orange (bell) pepper, cut into strips

1 medium carrot, cut into matchsticks

50 g/2 oz small seedless grapes

10 ml/2 tsp chopped coriander (cilantro)

15 ml/1 tbsp sesame seeds

15 ml/1 tbsp cold-pressed extra virgin olive oil

10 ml/2 tsp freshly squeezed lemon juice

5 ml/1 tsp tamari soy sauce

1 whole garlic clove

Sea salt (optional)

1 Place the rice and water in a large saucepan along with the cardamoms, cassia bark or cinnamon and lime leaves, if liked.

2 Cover tightly with a lid and bring to the boil, reduce the heat and cook for about 15 minutes, then remove from the heat and set aside for about 5 minutes with the lid still on.

3 Trim the green beans, then steam or boil them for about 3 minutes. Then, while they are still quite firm, drain and plunge immediately under cold water. Cut into 2 cm/¾ in pieces and put in a large salad bowl.

4 Place the onion and pepper in a bowl and pour boiling water over them. Leave for about 5 seconds (no longer). This will remove any harshness from their flavours. Drain and plunge immediately into cold water to crisp them up again. Dry on kitchen paper (paper towels), then chop quite finely and add to the salad bowl with the carrot matchsticks and the grapes.

5 Remove the cardamoms, cassia bark or cinnamon and lime leaves from the rice. (All the water should have been absorbed.) Spoon the rice into the salad bowl and add the chopped coriander and sesame seeds.

6 To make the dressing, put the olive oil, lemon juice and soy sauce in a small bowl. Add the juice of the garlic clove by crushing it carefully in a garlic press. Do not allow any of the solid matter to fall into the bowl.

7 Stir all the dressing ingredients together to combine them, then pour over the salad.

8 Toss the salad thoroughly to combine all the ingredients. Taste for seasoning and add a little more lemon juice or sea salt, if liked.

9 Set the salad aside for about 20 minutes to allow the flavours to develop.

Mediterranean Mixed Bean Salad

You don't have to have kombu seaweed to make this recipe successfully. I do think it's worth seeking out, however, so that you can keep a packet in your store cupboard for whenever you cook dried beans – the natural glutamic acid in kombu cuts down the cooking time of the beans and makes them much more digestible. Kombu, like other seaweeds, is now widely available from health food stores, and seaweed is considered to be one of the ultimate detox foods – cleansing, packed with vitamins and minerals, and a wonderful aid to digestion. You can use any mixture of beans you like in this recipe, but try to provide a range of colours, shapes and flavours. Remember, small beans will cook more quickly than large varieties, so adjust the cooking times accordingly.

SERVES 4

40 g/1½ oz kidney beans

40 g/1½ oz cannellini beans

40g/1½ oz chick peas (garbanzos)

40 g/1½ oz green continental lentils

1 strip of dried kombu (about 13 cm/5 in)

50 g/2 oz green beans

1 small red onion, finely chopped

1 small yellow or orange (bell) pepper, cut into chunks

25 black olives, stoned (pitted)

15 basil leaves

For the dressing:

30 ml/2 tbsp cold-pressed extra virgin olive oil

15 ml/1 tbsp fresh apple juice

10 ml/2 tsp cider vinegar

A few drops of freshly squeezed lemon juice

1 garlic clove, crushed

Freshly ground black pepper

Sea salt, to taste

1 Place the kidney beans, cannellini beans and chick peas in a bowl and cover with cold water. Soak for 8 hours, or overnight.

2 Drain and rinse the beans and chick peas, then place them in a large saucepan of fresh water with the kombu seaweed. Bring to the boil, remove any scum from the surface and boil for 10 minutes. Remove from the heat, drain and rinse.

3 Place the boiled beans, chick peas, kombu and lentils in a saucepan of fresh water, bring to the boil and simmer gently for 20–30 minutes until tender (the cooking time will vary according to the variety of bean and how recently they have been dried). Alternatively, after boiling for 10 minutes, simmer in a slow cook pot for about 2½ hours. (This is a good way to cook dried beans, because it is gentle and helps to retain their shape and texture, but they must have been boiled rapidly first.)

4 Drain the beans and discard the kombu (you can finely chop it into the salad if you like).

5 Bring a steamer to the boil and steam the green beans for 4 minutes until they are just tender, or boil them for about 3 minutes. Plunge them immediately under cold water, then cut them into 2 cm/¾ in pieces and put in a large salad bowl.

6 Add the onion and pepper to the salad bowl together with the olives and basil leaves.

7 Next make the dressing. Put the olive oil, apple juice, cider vinegar and lemon juice in a small bowl. Add the crushed garlic clove, then stir well to combine all the ingredients.

8 Test for seasoning, then add freshly ground black pepper and a little sea salt to taste.

9 Pour the dressing over the salad ingredients and toss carefully to coat and mix, avoiding breaking up the beans in the process.

10 Leave for about 20 minutes to allow the flavours to mellow before serving.

Potato Salad with Creamy Salad Dressing

Use Jersey Royals or any other salad potatoes with good flavour for this dish. Chives, spring onions (scallions) and parsley are all considered great detoxers, as is the dressing with its fresh fruit juice, cider vinegar and olive oil.

SERVES 4

---

1 kg/2¼ lb waxy salad potatoes, washed

A sprig of mint

30 ml/2 tbsp snipped chives or finely chopped spring onion (scallion)

15 ml/1 tbsp chopped parsley

375 ml/13 fl oz/1½ cups Creamy Salad Dressing (see page 112)

---

1 Bring a steamer to the boil, then add the potatoes with the sprig of mint and cook until just tender. Alternatively, place in a pan of rapidly boiling water and simmer until just tender, drain, then place the sprig of mint in the saucepan with the potatoes and shake briskly to bruise the mint against the potatoes.

2 Set the potatoes on one side to cool (do not remove the mint until completely cold).

3 Discard the mint and cut the potatoes into 2 cm/¾ in pieces, then place them in a salad bowl along with the chopped chives or spring onion and the parsley.

4 Add the Creamy Salad Dressing and toss all the ingredients well to combine. Set aside for at least 20 minutes to allow the flavours to mingle.

Creamy Salad Dressing

This dressing makes a perfect detox accompaniment to all kinds of salads and vegetables, particularly potatoes.

MAKES ABOUT 450 ML/¾ PT/2 CUPS

45 ml/3 tbsp cold-pressed extra virgin olive oil

30 ml/2 tbsp wholemeal rice flour

A pinch of English mustard powder

300 ml/½ pt/1¼ cups soya milk

1 whole garlic clove

5 ml/1 tsp tamari soy sauce

25 ml/5 tsp fresh apple juice

20 ml/4 tsp cider vinegar

2.5 ml/½ tsp freshly squeezed lemon juice

Freshly ground black pepper

Sea salt (optional)

1 Heat the olive oil in a frying pan (skillet), then carefully stir in the rice flour and mustard powder. Gradually add the soya milk, stirring continuously. Continue cooking and stirring until the mixture thickens.

2 Crush the garlic clove in a garlic press and add a few drops of the garlic juice to the pan. Do not allow any solid matter to fall into the pan.

3 Add the soy sauce and very carefully stir in the apple juice.

4 Slowly add the cider vinegar, stirring continuously to prevent the mixture curdling.

5 Stir in the lemon juice, then test for seasoning and add freshly ground black pepper, and a little sea salt, if liked.

6 Set the dressing aside to cool. As it cools, stir vigorously every now and again to prevent it congealing. If it seems to be getting too sticky, use a balloon whisk or fork to whisk in a little extra soya milk. Once cool, it should have a smooth, thick, pouring consistency.

Potato and Celery Salad with Olive Oil and Apple Juice Dressing

The dressing used here is a good all-purpose salad dressing, useful for virtually any salad mixture – and the olive oil, cider vinegar and fruit juices make it a great detoxer. Try using delicious pink fir apple potatoes for this recipe, though any flavoursome salad variety will work well.

SERVES 4
1 kg/2¼ lb salad potatoes, washed
A sprig of mint
30 ml/2 tbsp snipped chives or finely chopped spring onion (scallion)
15 ml/1 tbsp chopped parsley
3 celery sticks, chopped
A handful of celery leaves, chopped
20 basil leaves
120 ml/4 fl oz/½ cup Olive Oil and Apple Juice Dressing (see page 115)

1 Bring a steamer to the boil, then add the potatoes with the sprig of mint and cook until just tender. Alternatively, place in a pan of rapidly boiling water and simmer until just tender, drain, then place the sprig of mint in the saucepan with the potatoes and shake briskly to bruise the mint against the potatoes.

2 Set the potatoes on one side to cool (do not remove the mint yet).

3 Once the potatoes are cool, discard the mint and cut them into 2 cm/¾ in pieces. Place them in a salad bowl with the chives or spring onion and the parsley.

4 Add the chopped celery and celery leaves to the salad bowl.

5 Roughly tear the basil leaves and add these to the salad bowl.

6 Pour the dressing over the potato mixture and toss all the ingredients well to combine. Set aside for at least 20 minutes to allow the flavours to mingle.

Olive Oil and Apple Juice Dressing

MAKES ABOUT 175 ML/6 FL OZ/¾ CUP

100 ml/3½ fl oz/scant ½ cup cold-pressed extra virgin olive oil

30 ml/2 tbsp cider vinegar

30 ml/2 tbsp fresh apple juice

15 ml/1 tbsp tamari soy sauce

5 ml/1 tsp mild mustard

1 whole garlic clove

Freshly ground black pepper

Sea salt, to taste

1 Place the olive oil, cider vinegar, apple juice, soy sauce and mustard in a small bowl and stir thoroughly.

2 Crush the garlic clove in a garlic press and add a few drops of garlic juice to the dressing. Do not allow any of the solid matter to fall into the bowl. Stir well.

3 Test the dressing for seasoning, and add freshly ground black pepper and a little sea salt to taste.

Celery, Apple and Mixed Nut Salad

Apples and celery are excellent cleansers and are combined here with nuts to create a crunchy and satisfying salad dish. Make sure you use a really crisp, juicy apple: grainy or floury varieties really do not work for this recipe.

SERVES 4

50 g/2 oz/½ cup walnuts

50 g/2 oz/½ cup almonds or other nuts

4 celery sticks, chopped into 5 mm/¼ in pieces

1 small red onion, finely chopped

15 ml/1 tbsp freshly squeezed lemon juice

1 large or 2 small crisp red eating (dessert) apples, cored and sliced

30 seedless white grapes

10 basil leaves

2 handfuls of watercress, stems removed

100 ml/3½ fl oz/scant ½ cup Apple and Walnut Dressing (see page 117)

1 Taste the walnuts. If the skins are bitter, bring a small pan of water to the boil, and drop the walnuts into it. Leave for about 10 seconds.

2 Remove the walnuts with a slotted spoon, then rub them in a tea towel (dish cloth) to remove most of the skins. Alternatively, peel off the skins with your fingers.

3 Place the walnuts and almonds (or other nuts) in a large salad bowl.

4 Add the chopped celery and onion to the salad bowl.

5 Put the lemon juice in a shallow dish. Dip the apple slices in the lemon juice to prevent them discolouring. Add to the salad bowl.

6 Add the grapes, basil leaves and watercress sprigs to the salad bowl.

7 Pour the dressing over the salad and toss well to combine and coat all the ingredients.

Apple and Walnut Dressing

The warm, rich flavour of walnut oil marries wonderfully with the sweetness of the apple juice and the tang of cider vinegar in this dressing.

MAKES ABOUT 150 ML/¼ PT/⅔ CUP
60 ml/4 tbsp fresh apple juice
30 ml/2 tbsp walnut oil
30 ml/2 tbsp cold-pressed extra virgin olive oil
30 ml/2 tbsp cider vinegar
Freshly ground black pepper
Sea salt, to taste

1 Place the apple juice, oils and cider vinegar in a small bowl. Add freshly ground black pepper and stir thoroughly.

2 Test for seasoning and add a little sea salt, if liked.

FISH DISHES

Whatever sort of diet you're following, you can't go wrong with fish. It's healthy and remarkably quick to cook and with the accompaniments I've suggested, will satisfy the biggest appetite. Nowadays there are literally dozens of varieties available from your local supermarket or fishmonger. When buying fish, always choose the freshest you can – the flesh should be firm and the scales and eyes should look bright and shiny.

Beetroot, Orange and Fennel Sauce

This is a useful sauce for all kinds of rich-fleshed fish, such as herring, salmon and trout. Both the beetroot (red beet) and the orange juice remain uncooked in this sauce so they lose none of their goodness.

MAKES ABOUT 150 ML/¼ PT/⅔ CUP

1 raw medium beetroot, peeled and quartered

1 medium orange, peeled and quartered

15 ml/1 tbsp cold-pressed extra virgin olive oil

1 small onion, finely chopped

2.5 ml/½ tsp fennel seeds

2.5 ml/½ tsp celery seeds

10 ml/2 tsp buckwheat flour

2.5 ml/½ tsp cider vinegar

Freshly ground black pepper

1 Put the beetroot and orange pieces in a blender and blend for about 20 seconds until smooth and frothy, then press through a sieve (strainer). Alternatively, feed them through a juicer. Set the juice aside.

2 Heat the olive oil in a pan, and fry (sauté) the onion gently for about 1 minute, then add the fennel and celery seeds and continue cooking for a further minute.

3 Stir in the buckwheat flour and cook for 1 minute on a low heat, stirring continuously to prevent sticking.

4 Stir in the cider vinegar and 15 ml/1 tbsp of the prepared juice and continue cooking for about 1 minute.

5 Remove from the heat and gradually stir in the rest of the juice, then set the sauce on one side while you cook your choice of fish.

Tuna Steaks in a Hazelnut and Herb Crust

This is simple, quick and delicious. Ask your fishmonger to slice two thick steaks horizontally, so you end up with four thin pieces, or you can do it yourself with a sharp knife. The hazelnut (filbert) crust helps the fish stay moist and flavoursome during cooking. Serve with Savoury Vegetable Rice (see page 162) and a Mixed Green Salad (see page 89).

SERVES 4

Freshly squeezed juice of ½ large lemon

100 g/4 oz/1 cup hazelnuts

15 ml/1 tbsp chopped dill (dill weed)

15 ml/1 tbsp chopped parsley

5 ml/1 tsp chopped thyme

1 garlic clove, crushed

45 ml/3 tbsp cold-pressed extra virgin olive oil

550 g/1¼ lb fresh tuna steak

Lemon slices and sprigs of dill, to garnish

Freshly ground black pepper and a little sea salt

1 Pour the lemon juice into a blender with the nuts, herbs, garlic and 10 ml/2 tsp olive oil and blend until you get a fine crumb consistency.

2 Line a grill (broiler) pan with aluminium foil, then oil the foil with about 5 ml/1 tsp olive oil.

3 Place the tuna steaks on the foil. Pile a quarter of the nut mixture on top of each steak, then spread across the surface, pressing firmly into the fish so you gently flatten and spread the steak to a thickness of about 1 cm/½ in (no thinner, or it will dry out during cooking).

4 Season the steaks with pepper and a little sea salt. Finally, drizzle the remaining oil over the fish.

5 Grill (broil) carefully for about 5 minutes, until the topping is golden brown. The fish must be only just cooked so it is still quite moist and succulent.

6 Serve immediately, garnished with lemon slices and sprigs of dill.

Trout Fillets with Beetroot, Orange and Fennel Sauce

The sharpness of the orange and the sweetness of the beetroot (red beet) marry well with the rich flesh of trout. Trout, like all oil-rich fish, is an excellent addition to a detox diet.

SERVES 4

4 trout fillets

5 ml/1 tsp freshly squeezed lemon juice

50 g/2 oz/½ cup millet flakes

15 ml/1 tbsp cold-pressed extra virgin olive oil

Orange zest, to garnish

Beetroot, Orange and Fennel Sauce (see page 119), to serve

---

1 Sprinkle the fillets with lemon juice and then roll in the millet flakes, pressing the millet firmly into both sides of the fish to help it stick.

2 Heat the oil in a large pan (skillet) and fry (sauté) the fillets for about 3 minutes on each side.

3 Place the fish on individual plates and garnish with orange zest. Serve with a carefully poured pool of Beetroot, Orange and Fennel Sauce.

Monkfish Stir-fry

You can use monkfish, or huss which is cheaper. Both work well in stir-fries because their dense flesh holds together during cooking. They also have the distinct advantage of being boneless, so are ideal for folk who dislike fussing over bones. The single central cartilaginous bone is easy to deal with – I usually leave it in during cooking.

SERVES 4

---

45 ml/3 tbsp cold-pressed extra virgin olive oil

65 g/2½ oz fine green beans, trimmed

2 large celery sticks

1 medium carrot

A handful of celery leaves, chopped

1 red onion, finely chopped

1 medium courgette (zucchini), sliced

1 garlic clove, crushed

1 chilli, seeded and finely chopped

2 cm/¾ in piece of fresh root ginger, peeled and grated

300 g/11 oz moong bean sprouts

30 g/2 tbsp chopped dill (dill weed)

Freshly squeezed juice of ½ large lemon

450 g/1 lb monkfish or huss, skinned

15 ml/1 tbsp tamari soy sauce

Sprigs of coriander (cilantro), to garnish

1 Heat the olive oil in a wok or large, heavy frying pan (skillet).

2 Cut the beans into 2 cm/1 in pieces. Cut the celery and the carrot into 5 mm/¼ in thick sticks.

3 Stir-fry the beans, celery, carrot, celery leaves and onion for 3 minutes, then add the courgette, garlic, chilli and grated ginger.

4 Stir in the beansprouts, dill and lemon juice and continue cooking for 4 minutes.

5 Cut the fish into 3 cm/1¼ in pieces. Add to the stir-fry with the soy sauce and continue cooking for 4 minutes, until the fish is just tender.

6 Serve immediately, garnished generously with sprigs of coriander.

Mediterranean Fishcakes with Chargrilled Vegetables

You can use any kind of fish for this recipe, but I like to combine a richer fleshed variety, such as trout, with a more delicate white fish.

SERVES 4

For the Mediterranean Fishcakes:

400 g/14 oz potatoes, scrubbed

275 g/10 oz trout fillet

275 g/10 oz haddock fillet

15 ml/1 tbsp freshly squeezed lemon juice

Freshly ground black pepper

Sea salt

1 red (bell) pepper

45 ml/3 tbsp cold-pressed extra virgin olive oil

1 large onion OR 4–5 shallots, finely chopped

1 garlic clove, crushed

7.5 ml/1½ tsp chopped oregano

7.5 ml/1½ tsp chopped rosemary

25 ml/1½ tbsp chopped flatleaf parsley, plus a few leaves for garnish

60 ml/4 tbsp sesame seeds

For the Chargrilled Vegetables:

1 fennel bulb, chopped

1 red pepper, quartered

1 green pepper, quartered

2 red onions, roughly chopped

15 ml/1 tbsp cold-pressed extra virgin olive oil

15 ml/1 tbsp rice or potato flour

150 ml/¼ pt/⅔ cup well flavoured stock

1 First, make the fishcakes. Boil or steam the potatoes until tender. Drain and leave to cool.

2 Meanwhile, place the fillets of fish on a plate over a saucepan of water, or in a steamer. Sprinkle with the lemon juice, season with black pepper and a little sea salt, then steam until just tender.

3 Skin the pepper by holding it over a flame briefly until the skin chars and peels away from the flesh, then core and seed before finely chopping the flesh.

4 Heat 30 ml/2 tbsp olive oil in a frying pan (skillet), then gently cook the onion or shallots and the pepper until very soft but not coloured. Add the garlic and continue cooking for another 2 minutes. Add the herbs.

5 Drain the liquor from the cooked fish into the frying pan and continue cooking for another 4 minutes.

6 When the potatoes are cool, peel off the skins, place in a large bowl and mash with a fork or potato masher.

7 Gently lift the fish fillets from their skin, check for bones and finely flake the flesh. Add to the potato.

8 Carefully remove the pepper and onion mixture from the frying pan with a slotted spoon and add to the fish and potato. Reserve the liquor in the frying pan.

9 Mix together the fish, potato and pepper and onion mixture thoroughly and check the seasoning. Form 12 balls from the mixture and roll in the sesame seeds. Cover and leave in a cool place for at least 30 minutes.

10 To prepare the Chargrilled Vegetables, reheat the grill (broiler), drizzle the olive oil over the vegetables and grill (broil) until tender and well browned.

11 Meanwhile, heat the remaining 15 ml/1 tbsp olive oil in a clean frying pan and fry the fishcakes over a medium heat for about 15 minutes until crisp on both sides.

12 Immediately before serving, add the stock to the reserved fish cooking liquor, heat and then stir in the flour to thicken. Serve with the fishcakes and vegetables, garnished with flatleaf parsley.

Yoghurt and Dill Dressing

This pleasant creamy herb dressing is suitable for most fish.

MAKES ABOUT 150 ML/¼ PT/⅔ CUP

100 ml/3½ fl oz/ scant ½ cup goats', sheep's or soya yoghurt

2 large spring onions (scallions), finely chopped

20 ml/4 tsp tamari soy sauce

20 ml/4 tsp chopped dill (dill weed)

Freshly squeezed lemon juice, to taste

1 Place the yoghurt in a small bowl.

2 Add the chopped spring onions, soy sauce and dill.

3 Taste and add lemon juice to sharpen the dressing. If the yoghurt is very acidic, add only a drop or two of lemon juice. If the yoghurt is creamy and mild, add up to 15 ml/1 tbsp of lemon juice.

4 Stir the ingredients together thoroughly.

Sardines with Yoghurt and Dill Dressing

Sardines are quick and easy to clean providing you have a sharp knife, but handle the fish carefully as they are quite delicate. First remove the tail and head just below the gills. Then make a slit from the vent to the gills and remove the insides. With your fingers, rub from tail end to head end to loosen and remove scales, then rinse inside and out. The whole process does not take long.

SERVES 4

12–16 fresh or thawed frozen sardines, cleaned and scaled

2 spring onions (scallions), finely chopped

60 ml/4 tbsp fresh apple juice

15 ml/1 tbsp tamari soy sauce

15 ml/1 tbsp freshly squeezed lemon juice

Freshly ground black pepper

Yoghurt and Dill Dressing (see page 126), to serve

1   Arrange the cleaned sardines in a grill (broiler) pan and sprinkle the chopped spring onions over.

2   In a small jug or bowl, mix together the apple juice, soy sauce and lemon juice, then pour the mixture over the fish.

3   Season with freshly ground black pepper, then grill (broil) for 6–7 minutes, turning once.

4   Serve with a side dish of Yoghurt and Dill Dressing.

Speedy Swordfish Steaks with Lime, Basil and Coriander

I sometimes use tope, marlin or fresh tuna for this recipe – they all work equally well. Look and see what's good and cheap in the fishmonger. This is an excellent quick dish for when you're in a hurry.

SERVES 4

45 ml/3 tbsp cold-pressed extra virgin olive oil

4 swordfish steaks

30 ml/2 tbsp chopped coriander (cilantro)

1 red onion, finely chopped

½ fennel bulb, finely chopped

1 small carrot, finely chopped

1 garlic clove, crushed

175 g/6 oz broccoli florets

Freshly squeezed juice of 2 limes

6 basil leaves

350 g/12 oz cold cooked potatoes

Freshly ground black pepper

Sea salt

Lime slices, to garnish

1 Pour 15 ml/1 tbsp olive oil into a large grill (broiler) pan and coat the bottom.

2 Arrange the fish steaks in the pan.

3 Sprinkle the coriander, onion, fennel, carrot and garlic over the fish. Break the broccoli into tiny florets and add those to the pan.

4 Sprinkle the lime juice over the fish and vegetables, then roughly tear up the basil leaves and add these.

5 Thinly slice the cold cooked potato and add to the pan in a layer over the fish and vegetables.

6 Drizzle the remaining olive oil over, then season with black pepper and a little sea salt.

7 Cook for about 7 minutes, basting carefully, then push the potatoes off the fish, turn the steaks and vegetables and cook for a further 4 minutes, continuing to baste, until the fish is just cooked through and still moist.

8 Remove from the heat and serve immediately with a garnish of lime slices.

Mullet with Plum and Ginger Relish

I use grey mullet for this though you could use bream, and mackerel works well too. Remember to ask the fishmonger to scale the mullet if you don't want to do it yourself. It's an easy job (use the back of a large heavy knife and scrape from head to tail) but rather messy.

SERVES 4

---

5 firm but ripe red plums, stoned (pitted)

15 ml/1 tbsp tamari soy sauce

6 juniper berries

Sea salt

1 mullet, about 1.25 kg/2½ lb, or 2 small ones

Plum and Ginger Relish (see page 131)

---

1 Slice one of the plums and reserve for garnish. Place the other four in the blender. Whiz for about 10 seconds until smooth and frothy. Alternatively, feed them through a juicer.

2 Pour the puréed plums into a small bowl, then stir in the soy sauce and the juniper berries along with a little sea salt.

3 Rinse the mullet and scrape off any remaining scales. Place in a large, lidded ovenproof dish.

4 Pour the plum mixture over the mullet, cover tightly with a lid or foil, then cook in a preheated oven at 180°C/350°F/gas mark 4 for about 25 minutes.

5 Garnish the mullet with the reserved slices of plum and serve with a dish of the warm Plum and Ginger Relish.

Plum and Ginger Relish

*The balance of sweetness and sharpness in this relish
complements any rich-fleshed fish, such as mackerel, herring
or mullet.*

SERVES 4

15 ml/1 tbsp sunflower oil

1 small onion, finely sliced

1 small piece of fresh root ginger, peeled and grated

1 small carrot, grated

4 red plums, stoned (pitted) and finely chopped

100 ml/3½ fl oz/scant ½ cup water

15 ml/1 tbsp tamari soy sauce

5 ml/1 tsp mild clear honey

2.5 ml/½ tsp freshly squeezed lemon juice

Sea salt, to taste

1   Heat the oil in a pan and sauté the onion for 1 minute,
then add the grated root ginger and carrot to the pan,
stir and cook for a further minute.

2   Add the plums, water, soy sauce, honey and lemon
juice and continue cooking for a further 3 minutes.

3   Add a little sea salt, then taste for seasoning. If
necessary, stir in a little more honey and cook for a
moment or two longer.

4   Serve warm accompanying the fish of your choice.

Pan-cooked Spanish Fish and Vegetables

You can use any mixture of fish in this: cod, haddock, coley, tuna and huss all work well.

SERVES 4

---

45 ml/3 tbsp cold-pressed extra virgin olive oil

2 large onions, sliced

1 celery stick, chopped

1 large red (bell) pepper, seeded and chopped

1 courgette (zucchini), sliced

3 garlic cloves, crushed

1 small chilli, seeded and finely chopped

900 ml/1½ pts/3¾ cups good fish or vegetable stock

20 basil leaves, torn

10 ml/2 tsp chopped oregano

5ml/1 tsp chopped thyme

1 bay leaf

10 ml/2 tsp tamari soy sauce

450 g/1 lb potatoes, sliced

700 g/1½ lb mixed fish fillets

175 g/6 oz peas

20 black olives, stoned (pitted)

Salt and freshly ground black pepper

5 ml/1 tsp freshly squeezed lemon juice

Sprigs of flatleaf parsley, to garnish

1 Heat the olive oil in a large frying pan (skillet). Add the onion, celery, pepper and courgette and fry (sauté) gently until softened but not coloured.

2 Stir the crushed garlic and chopped chilli into the onion mixture. Continue cooking for a further 3 minutes.

3 Remove the vegetables from the pan with a slotted spoon and keep warm.

4 Put the fish or vegetable stock, herbs and soy sauce in the pan and bring to the boil. Reduce to a simmer.

5 Add the potato slices and cook for about 6 minutes.

6 Cut the fish fillets into bite-sized pieces and stir into the pan together with the peas. Cook gently for a further 2 minutes (do not boil rapidly, or the fish will toughen).

7 Stir the onion, celery and pepper mixture into the fish and potato, add the olives and cook for a further 1–2 minutes to heat through gently but thoroughly. Taste, adjust the seasoning and sharpen with a little lemon juice, if liked.

8 Serve garnished with generous sprigs of parsley.

Salmon Steaks with Orange, Watercress and Strawberries

The clean citrus flavour of the oranges marries well with the oil-rich salmon in this recipe. As with all detox dishes, it is important to use fresh ingredients wherever possible, so try to make your own orange juice for the dressing if you can. You will need 3–6 oranges (depending on size) to make 250 ml/8 floz/1 cup juice.

SERVES 4

---

4 salmon steaks

4 spring onions (scallions), finely chopped

250 ml/8 fl oz/1 cup freshly squeezed orange juice

20 ml/4 tsp tamari soy sauce

25 ml/5 tsp cold-pressed extra virgin olive oil

Freshly ground black pepper

15 ml/1 tbsp cider vinegar

2 oranges

8–10 strawberries

100 g/4 oz watercress

8 fine strips of orange zest

1   Arrange the salmon steaks in a flameproof dish and sprinkle the chopped spring onions over the fish.

2   Put 150 ml/¼ pt/⅔ cup of the orange juice in a small jug or bowl. Add 10 ml/2 tsp tamari soy sauce and 10 ml/ 2 tsp olive oil. Stir well to combine the ingredients, pour over the salmon steaks, then season the fish with freshly ground black pepper.

3   Place the fish under a medium-hot preheated grill (broiler) and cook for about 3 minutes per side, until the steaks have changed colour from deep rosy pink to pale pink, and the flesh flakes easily but is still succulent. Do not overcook. As soon as they are done, remove from the heat.

4   While the fish is cooking, prepare the salad dressing. Put the remainder of the orange juice, olive oil and soy sauce in a small jug or bowl with the cider vinegar and stir well.

5   Hull and halve the strawberries, or slice them if they are especially large, then peel and slice the oranges, removing any pips. Reserve four slices of orange and four strawberry halves or slices, then place the rest in a large bowl with the watercress.

6   Pour the salad dressing over the watercress salad, toss well and arrange around the outside of a large platter.

7   When the salmon steaks are cooked, transfer them carefully to the centre of the platter, spoon over any remaining cooking juices, then garnish with the reserved strawberry halves, orange slices and orange zest, and serve immediately.

POULTRY AND DAIRY DISHES

This section contains a range of main-course dishes that are not only healthy but delicious and satisfying too. And some, such as Chicken with Hazelnut, Orange and Herb Stuffing (see page 144), are just that little bit different and special, so you can enjoy a supper party with guests, without spoiling your detox routine.

Sweet Potato and Feta Bake

This is a wonderfully simple and sustaining supper dish.
Serve it with a big green salad.

SERVES 4
---

900 g/2 lb sweet potatoes, cut into chunks

450 g/1 lb potatoes, cut into chunks

15 ml/1 tbsp olive oil

225 g/8 oz/2 cups Feta cheese, crumbled

10 ml/2 tsp chopped thyme

10 ml/2 tsp chopped parsley

Freshly grated nutmeg

Freshly ground black pepper

Sprigs of parsley, to garnish

1 Steam or boil the sweet potatoes and potatoes until they are almost cooked, but still quite firm. Remove from the heat and slice.

2 Generously oil an ovenproof dish, then arrange half the sweet potatoes in the bottom. Sprinkle one third of the crumbled Feta over the top, then sprinkle one third of the herbs over and season with nutmeg and pepper.

3 Arrange the potatoes in a layer on top, add more cheese, herbs and seasoning.

4 Add another layer of sweet potato, more herbs and seasoning, then top with a layer of cheese.

5 Drizzle the remaining olive oil over the top, then cook in a preheated oven at 190°C/375°F/gas mark 5 for about 20 minutes, until crisp and brown and piping hot.

6 Garnish with sprigs of parsley before serving.

Spicy Chargrilled Chicken Breasts with Peppers and Rosemary

Rosemary, which adds fragrance and piquancy to this dish, is considered to be one of the best cleansing herbs. If you prefer only a gentle touch of chilli, remove the seeds before chopping it up. Try to prepare the marinade for this dish at least an hour in advance.

SERVES 4

Freshly squeezed juice of 1 large lemon

60 ml/4 tbsp cold-pressed extra virgin olive oil

25 ml/1½ tbsp fresh chopped rosemary

½–1 chilli, finely chopped

Sea salt and freshly ground black pepper

4 medium chicken breasts, skinned

1 large red (bell), pepper, roughly chopped

1 large green pepper, roughly chopped

3 red onions, quartered

Sprigs of rosemary, to garnish

1 Put the lemon juice into a large non-metallic dish with the olive oil, rosemary and chilli, and season with a little sea salt and freshly ground black pepper. Stir to combine the ingredients.

2 Make a series of diagonal slashes across the chicken breasts to allow the flavours to permeate, place in a shallow dish and pour over the marinade.

3 Add the chopped peppers and onions.

4 Stir to coat the chicken and vegetables, then cover and refrigerate for at least 1 hour.

5 Remove the chicken and vegetables from the marinade and arrange on a grill (broiler) pan. Pour the remaining marinade over them, then grill (broil) for about 5 minutes until the chicken is browned and the pepper slightly charred. Turn and cook the other sides.

6 Transfer to a warmed serving plate and serve immediately garnished with sprigs of rosemary.

Chinese Lemon Chicken

Thin slivers of lemon peel gently stir-fried with marinated chicken pieces create a rich and delicately aromatic sauce. Try to buy organic unwaxed lemons, but if these are not available, wash the lemon carefully before preparing it. Serve with Stir-fried Chinese Vegetables (see page 151) and rice.

SERVES 4

5 ml/1 tsp freshly squeezed lemon juice

10 ml/2 tsp cider vinegar

15 ml/1 tbsp fresh apple juice

15 ml/1 tbsp clear honey

2 cm/¾ in piece of fresh root ginger, peeled and grated

Freshly shredded zest of 1 lemon

4 spring onions (scallions), finely chopped

2 large or 3 small chicken breasts, skinned

900 ml/1½ pt/3¾ cups vegetable stock

400 g/14 oz rice noodles

30 ml/2 tbsp sesame oil

1 large green (bell) pepper, sliced

3 celery sticks, cut diagonally into 5 mm/¼ in wide slices

30 ml/2 tbsp tamari soy sauce

Lemon slices and coriander (cilantro) leaves, to garnish

1 First make the marinade. Put the lemon juice, cider vinegar, apple juice, honey, grated ginger, shredded lemon zest and chopped spring onion in a large bowl. Stir well to combine the ingredients.

2 Cut the chicken into 1 cm/½ in strips, then stir into the marinade and leave in a cool place for at least an hour.

3 Bring the stock to boiling point in a large pan and add the rice noodles. Cook for about 3 minutes, stirring occasionally.

4 When cooked, strain the noodles and toss in 10 ml/ 2 tsp sesame oil, then transfer to a warmed, covered dish.

5 Heat the remaining oil in a wok or large frying pan (skillet), then add the pepper and celery and stir-fry for about 1 minute.

6 Add the chicken and marinade and stir-fry for about 4 minutes, then add the soy sauce to the chicken mixture and cook for a further 1 minute.

7 Check that the chicken is cooked through, then transfer to a warmed serving dish and garnish with lemon slices and coriander leaves before serving with the rice noodles.

Paella

This delicious, subtly flavoured paella is made with round wholegrain rice, white fish, such as cod, and chicken. It might seem odd combining fish and meat in a single dish, but it's quite traditional in Spanish cooking, and works very well. Make sure you cook the rice thoroughly to achieve a thick, soft, creamy consistency.

SERVES 4

45 ml/3 tbsp cold-pressed extra virgin olive oil

2 medium red onions, finely chopped

1 yellow or orange (bell) pepper, chopped

2 tomatoes, chopped (optional)

3 fat garlic cloves, crushed

2 good-sized chicken breasts, skinned

10 ml/2 tsp paprika

350 g/12 oz/3 cups round wholegrain rice

A pinch of saffron powder (optional)

5 ml/1 tsp chopped rosemary

800 ml/1⅓ pts/3½ cups boiling water

1 additive-free stock (bouillon) cube

225 g/8 oz fresh or frozen peas

250 g/9 oz cod fillet, skinned and all bones removed

25 ml/1½ tbsp chopped flatleaf parsley

Parsley leaves, to garnish

1 Heat the olive oil in a large lidded pan. Add the onions, pepper and tomatoes, if using, and fry (sauté) them gently for about 4 minutes until soft.

2 Add the garlic and continue cooking gently for 2 minutes.

3 Cut the chicken breasts into 3 cm/1¼ in pieces and add to the pan with the paprika. Cook for a further 3 minutes, stirring occasionally and turning the chicken.

4 Add the rice, saffron and rosemary to the pan and continue cooking for about 4 minutes, stirring regularly.

5 Dissolve the stock cube in the boiling water, and pour into the pan. Cover and cook gently, stirring regularly, for about 35 minutes until the rice is tender and most of the liquid is absorbed.

6 Stir in the peas and continue cooking for 1 minute.

7 Cut the fish into 3 cm/1¼ in pieces and place carefully on top of the rice mixture and cover. Cook for a further 3 minutes over a very gentle heat, stirring the bottom of the pan if it seems likely to stick, but avoiding breaking up the fish. Add a very little extra water if it becomes too dry.

8 When the rice is completely cooked and the mixture creamy, remove from the heat and stir in the chopped parsley.

9 Serve immediately, garnished with a few leaves of flatleaf parsley.

Chicken with Hazelnut, Orange and Herb Stuffing

You will find that two large chicken breasts when filled with this substantial nutty stuffing will easily serve four people, especially when accompanied by a generous rice salad or a dish of rice noodles. For very large appetites, allow one chicken breast per person. Try to buy organic or at least free-range corn-fed meat.

SERVES 4

---

2 large chicken breasts

1 orange

1 small onion, chopped

50 g/2 oz/½ cup rice flakes

50 g/2 oz/½ cup hazelnuts (filberts)

1 garlic clove, crushed

10 ml/2 tsp freshly squeezed lemon juice

7.5 ml/1½ tsp chopped herbs, such as marjoram, thyme, rosemary

1 orange

Freshly ground black pepper

Sea salt

A little cold-pressed extra virgin olive oil

Sprigs of rosemary, to garnish

1 Beat the chicken breasts to flatten.

2 Grate the rind of half the orange and squeeze all the juice into a small bowl.

3 Put the grated rind and half of the juice into a food processor, with the remaining ingredients, except the olive oil, then process for about 10 seconds until thoroughly combined.

4 Check and adjust the seasoning, if necessary, then process briefly again.

5 Press half of the stuffing over each breast, then roll up and place in an ovenproof dish.

6 Drizzle the rest of the orange juice and a little olive oil over the chicken, and add a little more freshly ground black pepper.

7 Cover the dish with a lid or foil and bake the chicken in a preheated oven at 190°C/375°F/gas mark 5 for about 35 minutes.

8 Slice each breast in two, transfer to a heated platter and garnish with sprigs of rosemary before serving.

Piquant Vegetable and Feta Cheese Pie

This hearty winter supper dish is topped with flavoursome Greek sheep's cheese. The sharp lemony flavour of Feta allows you to use quite small quantities, but still achieve lots of flavour. Serve with a large green salad dotted with olives and tossed in a well flavoured olive oil dressing.

SERVES 4

2 large carrots, cut into chunks

450 g/1 lb unpeeled organic potatoes, cut into chunks

1 large parsnip, cut into chunks

45 ml/3 tbsp cold-pressed extra virgin olive oil

2 celery sticks, chopped

2 onions, chopped

1 red (bell) pepper, chopped

1 small chilli, seeded and chopped

5 ml/1 tsp chopped thyme

5 ml/1 tsp chopped parsley

10 ml/2 tsp roughly chopped basil leaves

450 ml/¾ pt/2 cups vegetable stock

1 large courgette (zucchini), thickly sliced

30 ml/2 tbsp buckwheat flour

100 g/4 oz/1 cup Feta cheese, crumbled

150 ml/¼ pt/⅔ cup sheep's, goats' or soya yoghurt

5 ml/1 tsp paprika

1 Steam or boil the carrots, potatoes and parsnip until just tender, then leave to cool.

2 Heat the olive oil in a large pan and fry (sauté) the celery, onion and pepper gently until softened but not coloured.

3 Stir the chilli into the onion mixture with the herbs. Continue cooking for a further 3 minutes.

4 Pour in the stock and continue cooking for about 15 minutes.

5 Add the courgette to the stock and continue cooking until the courgette is nearly tender.

6 In a small bowl, mix the buckwheat flour with enough water to make a paste. Stir the paste carefully into the stock and continue cooking for a couple more minutes, then remove from the heat and pour the mixture into a large ovenproof dish.

7 Slice the cooled potatoes, carrots and parsnips thickly and arrange them over the onion and courgette mixture.

8 Mix the crumbled Feta with the yoghurt and pour over the top of the sliced root vegetables.

9 Cook in a preheated oven at 190°C/375°F/gas mark 5 for about 20 minutes, until piping hot and golden brown on top.

10 Sprinkle with paprika before serving.

Conchiglie with Goats' Cheese and Green Beans

There is a good range of non-wheat pastas available in large supermarkets and health food stores these days. I like corn and vegetable conchiglie, but you can choose your own favourite shape and flavour, providing it is gluten-free.

SERVES 4

275 g/10 oz corn and vegetable conchiglie or other gluten-free pasta

350 g/12 oz green beans, trimmed

45 ml/3 tbsp cold-pressed extra virgin olive oil

1 large red onion, chopped

2 garlic cloves, crushed

40 black olives, stoned (pitted)

90 ml/6 tbsp chopped parsley

30 basil leaves

Freshly ground black pepper

200 g/7 oz goats' cheese

1 Cook the pasta in a large pan of boiling water according to the manufacturer's instructions. Do not overcook.

2 Steam or boil the green beans for about 4 minutes, then plunge them immediately in cold water to retain their crispness and colour, before draining and setting aside.

3 Heat the olive oil in a large frying pan (skillet) and fry (sauté) the onion and garlic gently until softened but not coloured. Stir in the olives, parsley, basil and green beans and continue cooking for about 1 minute. Remove from the heat.

4 Drain the pasta, then stir it into the onion, bean and olive mixture. Season with plenty of black pepper, then transfer to a flameproof dish.

5 Cut the goats' cheese into neat slices and arrange on top of the pasta mixture.

6 Place the dish under a preheated grill (broiler) and cook until the cheese begins to melt. Serve immediately.

VEGETABLE DISHES

The recipes I have chosen for this
section make the best of the huge
range of vegetables we can now buy.
They offer a wealth of colours, textures
and tastes – and, of course, vitamins!
Do buy organic vegetables wherever
possible – they are readily available in
large supermarkets and try to buy fresh
local produce when it is in season.
Don't be afraid to leave on the skins of
root vegetables such as potatoes,
parsnips and carrots – as long as they
are organic, they are very good for you,
so simply wash them and then slice or
chop as required.

Stir-fried Chinese Vegetables

This piquant vegetable dish makes a perfect accompaniment to Chinese Lemon Chicken (see page 140), but it can also be eaten as a main course if you double all the quantities, add a generous handful or two of cashew nuts or almonds and serve with rice noodles or rice. Moong bean sprouts are excellent additions to your detox diet. You can grow your own (see page 20) or buy them from the supermarket or health food store.

SERVES 4 AS A SIDE DISH

---

15 ml/1 tbsp sesame oil

½ chilli, seeded and finely chopped (optional)

2 cm/¾ in piece of fresh root ginger, peeled and grated

1 garlic clove, crushed

20 green beans, trimmed and cut into 2 cm/¾ in lengths

1 large carrot, cut into 5 mm/¼ in sticks

175 g/6 oz moong bean sprouts

100 g/4 oz pak choi (Chinese cabbage), coarsely shredded

15 ml/1 tbsp tamari soy sauce

5 ml/1 tsp freshly squeezed lemon juice

1 Heat the oil in a wok or large frying pan (skillet), then add the chilli, ginger and garlic and stir-fry for about 1 minute.

2 Add the beans and carrot and continue stir-frying for about 3 minutes.

3 Add the moong bean sprouts and pak choi and continue stir-frying for about 3 minutes.

4 Add the soy sauce and lemon juice and continue stir-frying for another 20 seconds before serving.

Vegetable Nut Crumble

This is a dish for hungry people. Use whatever vegetables are in season and if you have a glass ovenproof dish, arrange them in colour-contrasting layers. Be careful not to overcook the vegetables.

SERVES 4

450 g/1 lb organic potatoes, scrubbed and sliced

1 good-sized parsnip, scrubbed and sliced

225 g/8 oz carrots, scrubbed and sliced

75 g/3 oz green beans, trimmed

45 ml/3 tbsp cold-pressed extra virgin olive oil

1 medium leek, finely chopped

2 celery sticks, finely chopped

450 ml/¾ pt/2 cups vegetable stock

25 ml/1½ tbsp buckwheat flour

1 medium aubergine (eggplant), sliced

For the topping:

40 g/1½ oz/⅓ cup sunflower seeds

40 g/1½ oz/⅓ cup hazelnuts (filberts)

40 g/1½ oz/⅓ cup almonds

1 small onion, chopped

75 g/3 oz/¾ cup millet flakes

30 ml/2 tbsp chopped parsley

5 ml/1 tsp chopped thyme

5 ml/1 tsp chopped rosemary

15 ml/1 tbsp walnut oil

5 ml/1 tsp freshly squeezed lemon juice

15 ml/1 tbsp tamari soy sauce

A pinch or two of cayenne

Sprigs of rosemary, to garnish

1 Steam or boil the potato, parsnip and carrot slices with the green beans until par-cooked.

2 Heat 30 ml/2 tbsp olive oil in a pan and fry (sauté) the leek and celery gently until softened but not coloured.

3 Add the vegetable stock and continue to cook for about 4 minutes.

4 Put the buckwheat flour in a small bowl and add enough water to mix to a paste. Stir the paste into the stock and cook for about 4 minutes. Pour the mixture into a large ovenproof dish.

5 Heat the remaining oil gently in a large frying pan (skillet), add the aubergine slices and cook gently for about 3 minutes, then turn and cook the other side.

6 Arrange the slices of potato, parsnip, carrot, green beans and aubergine in layers on top of the leek and celery mixture.

7 Place all the crumble topping ingredients in a food processor and whiz for about 10 seconds to make a medium crumb consistency. Spoon the crumble topping over the vegetables, making sure you press it down around the edges.

8 Cook in a preheated oven at 180°C/350°F/gas mark 4 for about 20–25 minutes until the vegetables are just tender and the topping golden brown.

9 Garnish with sprigs of rosemary before serving.

Olive Oil Mash with Wilted Rocket Leaves

Olive oil mash is today's chic version of good old-fashioned British mashed potato. It is certainly a delicious and ideal way to serve potatoes while you are following a detox programme. In this recipe, a little swede (rutabaga) is added to give extra colour and sweetness, though you could use plain potato, or add sweet potato, parsnip, squash or pumpkin instead.

SERVES 4

---

750 g/1¾ lb organic potatoes, scrubbed and cut into chunks

225 g/8 oz swede, peeled and cut into chunks

60 ml/4 tbsp cold-pressed extra virgin olive oil

60 ml/4 tbsp soya milk

Freshly ground black pepper

Freshly grated nutmeg

1–2 drops freshly squeezed lemon juice

A handful of baby rocket leaves

Sea salt or herb salt, to taste

Sprigs of parsley, to garnish

1 Bring a steamer or a saucepan of water to the boil and steam or boil the potatoes and swede until tender.

2 Drain and transfer to a large bowl. Add the olive oil and soya milk, plenty of freshly ground black pepper, some freshly grated nutmeg and a few drops of fresh lemon juice. Mash vigorously until smooth and creamy.

3 Roughly tear up the rocket leaves and stir them into the mash.

4 Taste and add a little sea salt or herb salt, if necessary.

5 Transfer to a serving dish and garnish with sprigs of parsley before serving.

Rosemary and Orange Sauce

This sauce is good with many vegetable or fish dishes.

SERVES 4
15 ml/1 tbsp cold-pressed extra virgin olive oil
1 small onion, finely chopped
1 garlic clove, crushed
A pinch of cayenne
15 ml/1 tbsp tamari soy sauce
15 ml/1 tbsp freshly squeezed lemon juice
15 ml/1 tbsp rice flour
15 ml/1 tbsp chopped rosemary
Freshly squeezed juice of 2 good-sized oranges

1 Heat the oil in a pan and fry (sauté) the onion and garlic gently until softened but not coloured.

2 Stir in the cayenne, soy sauce and lemon juice.

3 Carefully stir in the rice flour and continue cooking for a further minute, stirring continuously.

4 Gradually stir in the rosemary and orange juice and continue cooking until the sauce thickens. If it seems too thick, add a little water.

Butternut Squash with Pine Nut and Leek Stuffing

A good recipe for using up leftover rice. Butternut squash are particularly good for this dish because the flesh remains firm when cooked. Onion squash also works well. Serve with Rosemary and Orange Sauce (see page 155)

SERVES 4

---

45 ml/3 tbsp cold-pressed extra virgin olive oil

1 medium leek, finely chopped

225 g/8 oz celeriac (celery root), grated

1 medium carrot, grated

400 g/14 oz/3½ cups cooked leftover round wholegrain rice

60 ml/4 tbsp pine nuts

15 ml/1 tbsp chopped rosemary

10 ml/2 tsp chopped thyme

30 ml/2 tbsp freshly squeezed lemon juice

A large pinch of cayenne

Sea salt, to taste

2 medium butternut squash, sliced lengthways and seeds removed

Sprigs of rosemary, to garnish

1 Heat the oil in a large frying pan (skillet). Finely chop the leek, add it to the pan and fry (sauté) gently for about 1 minute.

2 Stir the celeriac and carrot into the leek. Continue cooking for about 3 minutes.

3 Stir in the rice and pine nuts and continue cooking for about 2 minutes.

4 Stir in the herbs, lemon juice and cayenne and continue cooking for a further 1 minute.

5 Test for seasoning and stir in a little sea salt if necessary. Remove from the heat and set aside.

6 Meanwhile, arrange the squash halves in a roasting tray, cut side upwards.

7 Fill the squash with the pine nut stuffing, then carefully pour about 2 cm/¾ in water into the base of the roasting tray, cover the tray with aluminium foil and seal.

8 Cook in a preheated oven at 180°C/350°F/gas mark 4 for about 50 minutes, then check whether the squash is nearly tender. Remove the foil to crisp the stuffing, and cook for a further 15 minutes.

9 Garnish with sprigs of rosemary and serve with Rosemary and Orange Sauce.

Potato and Courgette Pancakes

Top these crispy pancakes with Thick Vegetable Sauce and Toasted Pine Nuts (see page 160), or crumble a little Feta cheese over the top and place under the grill (broiler) for a minute or two to brown.

SERVES 4

---

700 g/1½ lb organic potatoes, washed and coarsely grated

2 courgettes (zucchini), grated

1 large red onion, finely chopped

10 ml/2 tsp chopped oregano

10 ml/2 tsp freshly squeezed lemon juice

Freshly ground black pepper

Herb salt or sea salt

60 ml/4 tbsp cold-pressed extra virgin olive oil

Sprigs of rosemary or parsley, to garnish

---

1   Put the grated potatoes and courgettes into a large mixing bowl.

2   Add the chopped onion to the bowl together with the oregano, lemon juice, plenty of freshly ground black pepper and some herb or sea salt. Stir well to combine all the ingredients and set aside for about 10 minutes.

3   Heat 15 ml/1 tbsp oil in a non-stick frying pan (skillet).

4   Take about a quarter of the mixture and squeeze it hard between your hands to remove any excess moisture, then drop it in two portions into the hot oil, pressing it down to make two thick pancakes. Cook for about 4 minutes, or until very crisp, then carefully turn the pancakes over, press them down again and cook the other sides.

5 Remove the pancakes from the pan, place on a lightly oiled baking (cookie) sheet and transfer them to the oven to keep warm.

6 Wipe the pan clean, then repeat step 4 until you have eight pancakes.

7 Garnish with sprigs of parsley or rosemary and serve with a boat of Thick Vegetable Sauce with Toasted Pine Nuts.

Thick Vegetable Sauce with Toasted Pine Nuts

A useful sauce for pancakes, vegetable dishes or baked potatoes. You can also dilute the sauce with 450 ml/¾ pt vegetable stock or with soya or other non-dairy milk to make a tasty soup.

SERVES 4

¼ red (bell) pepper

15 ml/1 tbsp cold-pressed extra virgin olive oil

1 small onion, finely chopped

1 celery stick, finely chopped

1 medium carrot, finely chopped

2 sage leaves

5 ml/1 tsp chopped thyme

30 ml/2 tbsp rice flour

450 ml/¾ pt/2 cups well flavoured stock

10 ml/2 tsp freshly squeezed lemon juice

25 g/1 oz/¼ cup pine nuts

---

1 Place the pepper under a hot grill (broiler) until the skin starts to scorch. Turn the pepper until the skin is uniformly blackened all over. Place the pepper immediately in a polythene bag and seal it up. Leave it to cool for about 4 minutes.

2 Heat the oil in a pan, add the chopped vegetables, cover and cook very gently for about 4 minutes, removing the lid at intervals to stir them.

3 Rub the pepper in the polythene bag so that its charred skin flakes away from the flesh. Then remove it from the bag and scrape off any remaining skin, before chopping it up and adding it to the pan.

4 Stir in the sage, thyme and rice flour and continue cooking for 1 minute.

5 Stir in the stock and lemon juice and continue cooking for 3 minutes, until it thickens.

6 Pour the sauce into a food processor or blender and blend to a fairly smooth consistency, then pour back into the saucepan.

7 Place the pine nuts on a grill pan and grill (broil) until they just start to colour. Shake the pan and continue to cook for a few moments longer until golden brown.

8 Stir the pine nuts into the sauce and bring almost to the boil before serving.

Savoury Vegetable Rice

In this dish the vegetables are simply chopped and stirred uncooked into the herb-infused olive oil before being mixed with gently spiced wholegrain rice – a perfect detox dish. This is a very useful recipe, hot or cold. It can be eaten as a main course or if you omit the nuts it makes a good accompaniment to meat, fish or vegetable main dishes.

SERVES 2

175 g/6 oz/1½ cups round wholegrain rice

375 ml/13 fl oz/1½ cups water

2 cm/¾ in piece of cinnamon stick

2 bay leaves

1 sprig of rosemary

30 ml/2 tbsp cold-pressed extra virgin olive oil

1 garlic clove, crushed

10 ml/2 tsp tamari soy sauce

5 ml/1 tsp freshly squeezed lemon juice

10 ml/2 tsp chopped thyme

15 ml/1 tbsp chopped parsley

1 medium carrot, finely diced

50 g/2 oz baby sweetcorn (corn) cobs, sliced

50 g/2 oz broccoli, broken into tiny florets

½ red (bell) pepper, seeded and chopped

75 g/3 oz raw unsalted nuts – choose 1 or 2 from the following varieties: pine nuts, sunflower seeds, sesame seeds, hazelnuts (filberts), almonds, cashews

2–3 sprigs of rosemary, to garnish

1   Place the rice, water, cinnamon, bay leaves and sprig of rosemary in a large saucepan and bring to the boil. Reduce the heat to a simmer, cover tightly with a lid or foil and cook for about 15 minutes.

2   Remove the saucepan from the heat and leave, covered, for 5 minutes.

3   Meanwhile, heat the oil in a frying pan (skillet) and fry (sauté) the garlic gently for about 3 minutes until softened but not coloured. Turn off the heat and leave the oil to cool for a minute or two.

4   Stir the soy sauce and lemon juice into the garlic oil, then stir in the thyme and parsley.

5   Stir the carrot, sweetcorn, broccoli and pepper into the herb-infused oil.

6   Remove the cinnamon, bay leaves and rosemary sprig from the rice, then stir the rice into the vegetable mixture.

7   Place the nuts under a medium grill (broiler) and toast until they start to colour, then stir them into the rice mixture.

8   Serve garnished with a few sprigs of fresh rosemary.

Speedy Stir-fried Vegetables

Double the quantities of this recipe to make it into a quick main meal served with a big salad.

SERVES 4

250 g/9 oz fine rice noodles

2 carrots

8 baby sweetcorn (corn)

4 spring onions (scallions)

½ green (bell) pepper

4 Chinese leaves (stem lettuce)

100 g/4 oz firm tofu or home-made Tofu Cheese (see page 98)

30 ml/2 tbsp sesame oil

1 garlic clove, crushed

1 cm/½ in piece of fresh root ginger, peeled and grated

1 handful of mangetout (snow peas)

2 good handfuls of moong bean sprouts

1 Boil the noodles in a large pan of water for 3 minutes, then drain.

2 Cut the carrot into strips, about 1 cm/½ in wide and 5 mm/¼ in thick and the baby sweetcorn into 1 cm/½ in chunks. Slice the spring onions diagonally into 1 cm/½ in pieces. Core and seed the green pepper and cut it into 5 mm/¼ in strips. Cut the Chinese leaves into 1 cm/½ in diagonal slices.

3 Cut the tofu or Tofu Cheese into strips, about 1 cm/½ in wide and 5 mm/¼ in thick.

4 Heat the oil in a large frying pan (skillet) or wok, add the garlic and ginger and stir-fry for about 30 seconds.

5 Add the carrot, sweetcorn, spring onion, pepper and mangetout and continue stir-frying for 1 minute.

6 Add the Chinese leaves and continue stir-frying for a further minute.

7 Add the moong bean sprouts and tofu or Tofu Cheese and continue stir-frying for a further 2 minutes, taking care not to break up the tofu strips.

8 Toss in the noodles and serve.

Baked Beetroot in a Creamy Sauce

The best way to make this recipe is to bake the beetroot (red beet) in the oven, but that can be wasteful of energy if you are not cooking something else at the same time. Alternatively, steam or boil the beetroot in their skins and then simply finish the dish off in the oven. You can buy rice milk from health food stores, but if you have trouble obtaining it, use soya, goats' or nut milk.

SERVES 4

4 medium beetroot, scrubbed but not peeled

25 ml/5 tsp cold-pressed extra virgin olive oil

20 ml/4 tsp rice flour

300 ml/½ pt/1¼ cups rice milk

45 ml/3 tbsp chopped parsley

2.5 ml/½ tsp caraway seeds

1 spring onion (scallion), chopped

2.5 ml/½ tsp freshly squeezed lemon juice

Sea salt

Sprigs of parsley and a sprinkling of paprika, to garnish

1 Dry the beetroot with kitchen paper (paper towels), then rub 5–10 ml/1–2 tsp olive oil over the skins.

2 Place them in an ovenproof dish, cover and cook in a preheated oven at 160°C/325°F/gas mark 3 for about 2 hours, or until they are tender.

3 When they are cooked, remove from the oven, mop any remaining oil from the dish and leave the beetroot until cool enough to handle.

4 Peel off the skins, then arrange them back in the dish.

5 Heat 15 ml/1 tbsp olive oil in a pan. Add the rice flour and gradually stir in the rice milk. Continue cooking and stirring until the sauce thickens.

6 Stir in the parsley, caraway seeds and spring onion and cook for a further minute.

7 Season with lemon juice and a little sea salt, then pour over the beetroot. Return the beetroot to the oven and cook for about 15 minutes.

8 Serve garnished with sprigs of parsley and a sprinkling of paprika.

Carrots with Coriander and Nutmeg

Make sure you don't overcook the carrots; they should still have plenty of bite left in them.

SERVES 4

---

350 g/12 oz carrots, sliced

15 ml/1 tbsp cold-pressed extra virgin olive oil

1 garlic clove, crushed

15 ml/1 tbsp chopped coriander (cilantro)

A little freshly grated nutmeg

Sea salt or herb salt, to taste

Sprigs of coriander, to garnish

1 Steam or boil the carrots until they are only just tender (test them frequently with a fork).

2 Heat the oil in a frying pan (skillet) and fry (sauté) the garlic for about 2 minutes, taking care not to let it colour. Turn off the heat and remove all but the smallest fragments of garlic from the oil.

3 Drain the carrots, then add them to the frying pan along with the chopped coriander and a little freshly grated nutmeg.

4 Toss well to coat the carrots and mix the ingredients.

5 Test for seasoning and add a little sea salt or herb salt, if necessary.

6 Transfer to a warmed serving dish and garnish with sprigs of coriander.

Leeks and Courgettes Dressed with Herbs

A bright green dish of summer vegetables gently flavoured with English herbs. Crumble Feta or goats' cheese over the dish and grill (broil) briefly to make a light supper for two.

SERVES 4

15 ml/1 tbsp cold-pressed extra virgin olive oil

1 medium leek, sliced

1 courgette (zucchini), sliced

60 ml/4 tbsp water

15 ml/1 tsp chopped parsley

15 ml/1 tbsp chopped marjoram

Freshly ground black pepper

Herb salt or sea salt, to taste

1 Heat the oil in a large frying pan (skillet). Add the leek and courgette, cover and fry (sauté) gently for about 2 minutes, stirring occasionally to ensure that the slices do not colour.

2 Add the water and continue to cook, uncovered, for about 2 minutes.

3 Stir in the herbs and season with pepper, then continue cooking, uncovered, for a further minute. By this time the liquid should have all but disappeared and the vegetables should be just tender.

4 Test for seasoning and stir in a little more pepper and some herb or sea salt if necessary.

5 Transfer to a warmed serving dish and serve.

DESSERTS AND BAKING

Following a detox diet doesn't mean you can't have little treats now and then – desserts can be both healthy and delicious, as these recipes show. As well as the fruit puddings you might expect, there is also Cinnamon Rice Pudding (see page 175) for lovers of 'nursery' food; and if you are a reformed chocoholic, try Carob-coated Pears (see page 182) for a scrumptious alternative. This section also contains useful basic recipes for Home-made Yoghurt (see page 171) and Detox Loaf (see page 186) – so you can still enjoy a sandwich or a piece of toast!

Home-made Yoghurt

A bowl of creamy live yoghurt, along with some stewed fruit or a drizzle of honey is the simplest of detox desserts, and an excellent addition to your detox programme. It is easy to make your own non-dairy yoghurt, but do make sure all your utensils are scrupulously clean before you start and thoroughly rinsed of any detergent. Use live cows' milk yoghurt as a 'starter' if necessary – once your own non-dairy yoghurt gets going, you can then save some from each batch to make the next one. Some live commercial yoghurts are much richer sources of yoghurt culture (benign bacteria which convert the milk to yoghurt) than others. You may need to experiment to find an effective brand. If your final result is very thin, try leaving it a little longer, or strain it through a fine sieve (strainer). Don't waste the resulting liquid – use it to make a refreshing yoghurt drink mixed with some fresh fruit juice. You can use a wide-mouthed vacuum flask to make yoghurt; just make sure you can clean it easily.

MAKES ABOUT 600 ML/1 PT/2½ CUPS

600 ml/1 pt/2½ cups goats' or non-dairy milk

45 ml/3 tbsp live unsweetened yoghurt

1–2 drops of vanilla essence (extract), to taste

10 ml/2 tsp almond oil (optional)

1 Bring the milk to the boil, then cool to 50°C/165°F or until it feels only just comfortable when you dip in an (extremely clean) finger.

2 Stir in the yoghurt and taste. If it has a slightly 'beany' flavour that you don't like, add 1–2 drops vanilla essence.

3 Cover and leave in a warm place for about 8 hours, or until set.

4 When set, stir in the almond oil, if liked. This helps to give the yoghurt a creamier taste and texture.

Strawberry, Kiwi and Orange Cup

Kiwi fruit are excellent for a detox diet – they are cleansing, succulent, juicy and vitamin-packed, and have an excellent balance of acidity and sweetness. They create a stunning colour contrast of brilliant green against the rosy red of the strawberries in this quick and easy dessert.

SERVES 4

---

450 g/1 lb ripe strawberries, hulled

4 ripe kiwi fruit, peeled

200 ml/7 fl oz/scant 1 cup freshly squeezed orange juice

15–30 ml/1–2 tbsp honey or pure fruit juice concentrate

Sprigs of mint

1 Juice one of the kiwi fruit and two strawberries and add the orange juice. Test for sweetness and add honey or fruit juice concentrate if necessary.

2 Halve the remaining strawberries, or slice them if they are large, and slice the remaining kiwi fruit, removing the centre cores if they seem woody.

3 Place the fruit in a serving dish, and add two or three sprigs of mint.

4 Pour the juice over the fruit, stir gently and cover.

5 Refrigerate for about an hour.

6 Immediately before serving, remove the sprigs of mint from the fruit salad and discard, then decorate the dish with one or two fresh sprigs.

Spiced Baked Bananas

You should eat bananas that are very ripe while you are on a detox diet – keep them until their yellow skins are generously freckled with little brown spots and no green. Then the flesh inside will be soft and yellow, sweet and easy to digest. Bananas and their relatives, plantains, are used widely in India to soothe inflamed stomachs, and they are also a good source of toxin-eliminating pectin.

SERVES 4

Freshly squeezed juice of 1 lemon

....

30 ml/2 tbsp walnut oil

....

15–30 ml/1–2 tbsp clear organic honey

....

15 ml/1 tbsp goats' or soya milk

....

2.5 ml/½ tsp ground cinnamon

....

4 large ripe bananas, peeled

....

100 g/4 oz/1 cup chopped mixed nuts

....

1 Put the lemon juice, walnut oil, honey, milk and cinnamon into a small bowl and stir to combine.

2 Put the bananas in a baking dish and pour the lemon mixture over.

3 Sprinkle the nuts over the bananas.

4 Cover the dish with a lid or foil, then bake in a preheated oven at 180°C/350°F/gas mark 4 for about 45 minutes until the bananas are soft and syrupy and the nuts golden brown.

Baked Pears with Nutmeg

Pears are considered to be amongst the best detox fruit. Here, they are baked with a golden crust of rice and almonds flavoured with freshly grated nutmeg and vanilla. Make sure you use only pure vanilla essence (extract), not artificial vanilla flavouring.

SERVES 4

---

30 ml/2 tbsp round wholegrain rice

25 g/1 oz/¼ cup unblanched almonds

2 ml/⅓ tsp freshly grated nutmeg

A few drops of pure vanilla essence

175 ml/6 fl oz/¾ cup fresh apple juice

15 ml/1 tbsp sweet almond oil

5 ml/1 tsp clear organic honey (optional)

2 large ripe pears, peeled, halved and cored

1 Place the rice and almonds in a blender and blend until you obtain a medium-fine consistency. If your blender will not grind up rice or nuts, use ready-prepared ground rice and almonds, though these will not be wholegrain.

2 Transfer to a medium mixing bowl and add the grated nutmeg and the vanilla essence.

3 Add 30 ml/2 tbsp of the apple juice to the rice and almond mixture and set aside the rest of the juice.

4 Add the sweet almond oil to the mixture and stir to combine all the ingredients. Test for sweetness. If necessary, add 5 ml/1 tsp clear honey and stir.

5 Stuff the centres of the pears with the rice mixture, spreading a thin layer over the whole cut surface of each pear half.

6   Arrange the pears in an ovenproof dish, pour over the remaining apple juice, cover with a lid or foil and bake in a preheated oven at 180°F/375°F/gas mark 4 for about 50 minutes until the pears are soft and the topping crisp and golden brown.

Cinnamon Rice Pudding

Slowly cook this pudding until it turns a glorious caramel colour and is topped with a glistening dark brown skin. Serve hot or cold, by itself, or with fresh fruit sauce. Notice that you add rather more liquid than you normally would for a rice pudding – wholegrain rice always absorbs more than the white variety. If you have a sweet tooth, use a little more honey than stated.

SERVES 4

750 ml/1¼ pt/3 cups goats', or other non-dairy milk

10 ml/2 tsp almond oil

50 g/2 oz/½ cup round wholegrain rice

15 ml/1 tbsp clear honey

½ tsp grated lemon or orange zest

2.5 cm/1 in piece of cinnamon stick or 5 ml/1 tsp ground cinnamon

A few drops of vanilla essence (extract)

1   Pour the milk and almond oil into a medium to large ovenproof dish. Stir in the rice, honey, lemon or orange zest, cinnamon and vanilla essence.

2   Bake in a preheated oven at 150°C/300°F/gas mark 2 for 2½–3 hours, stirring once after the first hour, until the pudding has a thick, creamy consistency and the rice is very tender.

Harlequin Poached Pears

This is a very pretty dessert. The delicately pink and white striped pears are served with raspberries in a brilliant pool of fabulously rich fruit juice.

SERVES 4

250 ml/8 fl oz/1 cup fresh apple juice

350 g/12 oz raspberries

10 ml/2 tsp clear organic honey

2.5 cm/1 in piece of cinnamon stick

4 medium Williams pears

60 ml/4 tbsp thick goats', sheep's or soya yoghurt

2.5 ml/½ tsp ground cinnamon

1 Put the apple juice into a measuring jug.

2 Blend 175 g/6 oz raspberries in a blender, then add the purée to the measuring jug.

3 Top up with water to make 750 ml/1¼ pts/3 cups liquid. Add the honey and stir. Pour into a large saucepan and add the cinnamon stick.

4 Carefully pare even strips of peel down the length of the pears, leaving strips of skin in between to give a striped appearance. Leave the stalks intact.

5 Place the pears in the saucepan of juice, bring to the boil and simmer gently for 1–1¼ hours until the pears are tender and the juice has reduced to about 100 ml/3½ fl oz/scant ½ cup. During cooking, turn the pears regularly in the liquor so each part of the surface area is submerged for a time.

6 When cooked, remove the pears from the saucepan, reserving the liquor. Carefully pare off the remaining peel from the pears to reveal pink and white stripes.

7 Arrange the pears upright on individual plates. Add a spoonful of raspberries and strain the cooking liquor over the raspberries.

8 Add a dollop of thick yoghurt to each plate with a sprinkling of cinnamon to decorate.

Summer Fruits Crumble

This is a delicious way to use summer fruits. Test for sweetness as you gradually add the honey – the amount you need will depend upon the sweetness and ripeness of the fruit.

SERVES 4

275 g/10 oz mixed summer fruits such as strawberries, raspberries, stoned (pitted) cherries, red currants, blackcurrants, elderberries, blackberries

15 ml/1 tbsp water

60 ml/4 tbsp mild clear honey

75 g/3 oz/¾ cup almonds

75 g/3 oz/¾ cup millet flakes

25 g/1 oz/¼ cup wholemeal rice flour

45 ml/3 tbsp almond oil

Thick plain yoghurt, to serve

1 Put the summer fruits and water into a medium bowl and stir in 30 ml/2 tbsp honey. Test for sweetness and add a further 15–30 ml/1–2 tbsp honey if the fruit is still too sharp. Transfer to an ovenproof dish.

2 Place the almonds, millet flakes, rice flour and almond oil in a blender and blend for about 20 seconds to create a fine crumb consistency. If the mixture is too sticky to create a fine crumb, add a little more rice flour and blend again for a few seconds.

3 Sprinkle the crumble topping over the summer fruits, ensuring that it covers right to the edge of the dish. Press down slightly.

4 Cook in a preheated oven at 180°C/350°F/gas mark 4 for about 25 minutes, until the topping is golden brown and the fruit piping hot, then serve with thick creamy yoghurt.

Fresh Peach and Maple Syrup Sorbet

Maple syrup should only be eaten in strict moderation during a detox diet. Try to find the sweetest, ripest peaches in order to limit the amount of sweetening needed and test the fruit purée as you add the maple syrup to make sure you use as little as possible – remember if the sorbet is too sweet, it will lose its refreshing quality.

SERVES 4

8 sweet ripe peaches

15–45 ml/1–3 tbsp pure maple syrup

5 ml/1 tsp freshly squeezed lemon juice

Almond and Rice Fingers (see page 183), to serve

1   Set two peaches aside, then quarter and stone (pit) the rest and place them in a blender with 15 ml/1 tbsp maple syrup and the lemon juice. Blend to a purée. Taste and add more maple syrup if necessary, then blend again to a smooth consistency.

2   Pour the purée into a non-metallic container and put it in the coldest part of the freezer.

3   When the purée has frozen completely, remove from the freezer and plunge the container into a basin of very hot water, to release the frozen purée.

4   Place in a food processor or blender and process until it forms a fine granular consistency.

5   Return the purée to the non-metallic container and refreeze it.

6   Stone and slice the remaining two peaches. Spoon the sorbet into individual glass dishes, decorate with the peach slices and serve with Almond and Rice Fingers.

Luxury Fruit Salad

This is a gorgeous fruit salad. Vary the fruit to include your own favourites, but try to maintain a good contrast of colours and textures.

SERVES 4

2 oranges, peeled and quartered

3 fresh apricots, stoned (pitted) and quartered

Freshly squeezed juice of 1 lime

1 large ripe banana, peeled and sliced

8–10 lychees, peeled and stoned

8–10 ripe strawberries, hulled and quartered

2 kiwi fruit, peeled and sliced

1 medium mango, peeled

1 Place the oranges and apricots in a blender and blend to a smooth consistency. Add the lime juice to the mixture. Alternatively, feed the oranges, apricots and lime through a juicer.

2 Pour the orange, apricot and lime juice mixture into a large bowl.

3 Add the prepared banana, lychees, strawberries and kiwi fruit.

4 Cut the mango flesh away from the stone (pit). Chop it into neat pieces and add to the fruit salad.

5 Stir the ingredients together and set aside in a cool place for about ½–1 hour before serving.

Creamy Vanilla Sauce

This is a recipe for detox custard. It's excellent with fruit salads and stewed fruits, but eat it only in moderation. Make sure you use pure vanilla essence (extract), not artificial flavouring.

MAKES ABOUT 400 ML/14 FL OZ/1¾ CUPS

60 ml/4 tbsp sweet almond oil

30 ml/2 tbsp rice flour

300 ml/½ pt/1¼ cups soya milk

15 ml/1 tbsp mild clear honey

A few drops of vanilla essence

1 Put the almond oil in a medium saucepan and heat.

2 Reduce the heat, carefully stir in the rice flour and cook very gently for about 30 seconds.

3 Gradually stir in the soya milk, taking care not to let the mixture go lumpy or burn, and simmer gently for about 1 minute, stirring as it cooks.

4 When the sauce is thickened, stir in the honey and vanilla essence.

5 Serve hot or cold.

Carob-coated Pears

Carob sauce is excellent hot or cold with stewed pears, citrus fruits and bananas. Here it is used to create a tempting glossy coating for fresh pears.

SERVES 4

---

60 ml/4 tbsp sweet almond oil

60 ml/4 tbsp rice flour

450 ml/¾ pt/2 cups soya milk

50 g/2 oz/½ cup carob powder

30 ml/2 tbsp mild clear honey

A few drops of vanilla essence (extract)

4 ripe pears, peeled, halved and cored

A few flaked (slivered) almonds for decoration

---

1 Put the almond oil in a saucepan and heat gently.

2 Reduce the heat, carefully stir in the rice flour and cook very gently for about 30 seconds, then very gradually add about half of the soya milk, stirring continuously to prevent it going lumpy.

3 Remove from the heat and gradually whisk in the carob powder (use a balloon whisk), taking care not to let the mixture go lumpy. Then stir in the rest of the soya milk.

4 Return to the heat and simmer very gently for 1–2 minutes, stirring all the time, then stir in the honey and vanilla essence.

5 Pat the pear halves dry with kitchen paper (paper towels) and place flat side down on individual plates.

6 Pour the sauce over the pears so that they are completely coated, leave in a cool place for about 1 hour, then sprinkle with almond flakes and serve with a little jug of the remaining sauce.

Almond and Rice Fingers

These shortbread-style biscuits are delicious with fruit salads, sorbets and fruit creams. Alternatively, serve them with Fresh Apricot Sauce (see page 184) or Apricot and Almond Topping (see page 185). They are quite rich, so don't eat too many too often while you are on a detox plan. Make sure, incidentally, that you use gluten-free flour – this is now quite widely available in large supermarkets and in health food stores.

MAKES 10 SLICES

75 g/3 oz/¾ cup almonds

100 g/4 oz/1 cup rice flour

50 g/2 oz/½ cup gluten-free flour

45 ml/3 tbsp sweet almond oil

45 ml/3 tbsp mild clear honey

1 Place the almonds and the flours in a food processor and process for about 15 seconds until the almonds are finely ground. Gradually add the oil and honey, processing the mixture as you go.

2 Line a baking (cookie) sheet with baking parchment and brush with oil, then spread the mixture over the sheet, and press it down to a thickness of about 1 cm/ ½ in. Press around the edges of the mixture to make a neatly edged rectangle.

3 Bake in a preheated oven at 160°C/325°F/gas mark 3 for about 15–20 minutes, until golden brown.

4 Remove from the oven and leave to cool on the baking sheet for about 10 minutes. Then cut neatly into about 10 slices, or 6 rectangles if you are using it to make individual bases for a dessert with Fresh Apricot Sauce or Apricot and Almond Topping.

Fresh Apricot Sauce

Serve this sauce immediately it is made. You may find it is thick enough to spread over the top of the almond fingers. If not, serve it in little glass dishes with the biscuits alongside.

SERVES 4–6

450 g/1 lb ripe apricots, halved and stoned (pitted)

45–60 ml/3–4 tbsp mild clear honey or pure maple syrup

Almond and Rice Fingers (see page 183), to serve

1 Place the apricots in a blender with the honey or maple syrup, and blend for about 10 seconds, until smooth and creamy.

2 Test for sweetness. If necessary add another 15 ml/ 1 tbsp honey or maple syrup and blend for a few seconds more.

3 Serve immediately with Almond and Rice Fingers.

Apricot and Almond Topping

This is good not only on Almond and Rice Fingers (see page 183), but also as filling for sweet pancakes, and for spreading on rice cakes or crisply toasted slices of Detox Loaf (see page 186). Ideally, use unsulphured dried apricots and lemon zest from unwaxed, organic fruit.

SERVES 4–6

---

100 g/4 oz/⅔ cup dried apricots

150 ml/¼ pt/⅔ cup fresh apple juice

A small piece of lemon zest

50 g/2 oz/½ cup almonds

---

1 Put the apricots in a bowl and cover with water. Leave to soak for 8 hours or overnight.

2 Drain the fruit and discard the water. Place the apricots in a saucepan with the apple juice and lemon zest and bring to the boil. Reduce to a simmer and cook until the fruit are tender, about 10 minutes.

3 Set the pan aside to cool for about 5 minutes, then put the fruit and any remaining syrupy liquor in a blender with the almonds.

4 Blend for about 15 seconds to a smooth thick cream.

Detox Loaf

This loaf is made without wheat, yeast or sugar and is sweetened very lightly with fresh apple juice. Make sure you use potassium-based baking powder (available from health food stores) as this keeps the sodium content of the bread to a minimum. Gluten-free flour is available from health food stores, and increasingly these days from supermarkets. This loaf is especially good when sliced thinly and toasted, but remember you should not eat too much of it when you are on a detox diet, and you shouldn't spread butter on it.

MAKES 1 LOAF
450 g/1 lb gluten-free flour
10 ml/2 tsp cream of tartar
10 ml/2 tsp potassium-based baking powder
5 ml/1 tsp olive oil plus extra for oiling
150 ml/¼ pt/⅔ cup fresh apple juice
400 ml/14 fl oz/1¾ cups water
Sea salt

1 Place the flour, cream of tartar and baking powder in a large mixing bowl and stir thoroughly.

2 Add the olive oil, apple juice and water and stir to make a smooth batter.

3 Stir in a little sea salt, if liked.

4 Pour the batter into an oiled loaf tin (pan) and bake in a preheated oven at 190°C/375°F/gas mark 5 for about 40–50 minutes. Test the centre with a skewer. The loaf is cooked if it comes out cleanly. If batter sticks to the skewer when it is removed, continue cooking for 5–10 minutes.

5 Turn out on to a wire rack and cool thoroughly before slicing the loaf.

INDEX

fruit bowl 44
juices 14, 52–7
luxury fruit salad 180
nutty muesli 45
preparation 12, 24, 27
speedy snacks 29
summer fruits crumble 178
superfoods 16
sweetness 13
and yoghurt 29
see also specific fruits
fruity coleslaw 90

galettes stuffed with tuna and
  sweetcorn 46–7
garbanzos see chick peas
garlic 16
ginger 16
  ginger and lime wake-up 39
  mango, apple and ginger kick-start 53
  mixed melon starter 70–1
  plum and ginger relish 130, 131
gluten-free foods 19
grains 18–19
  see also millet; rice
grapefruit
  pink citrus 55
  toasted grapefruit and pineapple with
    almonds 42
grapes
  California salad with citrus dressing 92
  cucumber and grape juice 57
  fragrant rice salad 106–7
  grape and papaya juice 56
  melon and grape juice 54
green salad, mixed 89

haddock
  Icelandic beetroot and haddock
    salad 100–1
  Mediterranean fishcakes with
    chargrilled vegetables 124–6
  pan-cooked Spanish fish and
    vegetables 132–3
  Thai fish soup 64–5
harlequin poached pears 176–7
hazelnuts
  chicken with hazelnut, orange and
    herb stuffing 144–5
  hazelnut and lemon butter 79
  olive, pepper and hazelnut pâté 82–3
  tuna steaks in a hazelnut and herb
    crust 120–1
health advice 5
health supplements 23
herbal teas 14
herbs 22, 27
  chicken with hazelnut, orange and
    herb stuffing 144–5

crudités with creamy tofu dip 78–9
  feta, olive and summer herb
    salad 96–7
  leeks with courgettes dressed with
    herbs 169
  mixed green salad 89
  tuna steaks in a hazelnut and herb
    crust 120–1
  see also specific herbs
home-made yoghurt 171
hummus with crudités 80–1
hunger 7
huss
  pan-cooked Spanish fish and
    vegetables 132–3
  stir-fry 122–3

Icelandic beetroot and haddock salad
  with mustard dressing 100–1

kiwi fruit
  luxury fruit salad 180
  strawberry, kiwi and orange cup 172
kombu
  hummus with crudités 80–1
  Mediterranean mixed bean
    salad 108–10

laver
  nori maki 76–7
  Welsh breakfast 50–1
leeks
  butternut squash with pine nut and
    leek stuffing 156–7
  leeks with courgettes dressed with
    herbs 169
  vegetable salad with leeks, celeriac
    and broad beans 104–5
lemons 16
  Chinese lemon chicken 140–1
  citrus dressing 93
  hazelnut and lemon butter 79
  lemon zester 38
  papaya and citrus breakfast 41
  tofu, parsley and lemon dressing 105
limes
  ginger and lime wake-up 39
  papaya and citrus breakfast 41
  rice and cashew nut salad with lime
    dressing 94–5
  speedy swordfish steaks with lime,
    basil and coriander 128–9
linseed 23
luxury fruit salad 180
lychees, luxury fruit salad 180

mandarins
  beetroot and mandarin juice 56
  pink citrus 55